D0409959

ROSACEA

ROSACEA
DIAGNOSIS AND MANAGEMENT

WITH A CONTRIBUTION BY JONATHAN WILKIN

FRANK C. POWELL
Mater Misericordiae Hospital
Dublin, Ireland

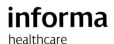

informa
healthcare

New York   London

Informa Healthcare USA, Inc.
52 Vanderbilt Avenue
New York, NY 10017

© 2009 by Informa Healthcare USA, Inc.
Informa Healthcare is an Informa business

No claim to original U.S. Government works
Printed in the United States of America on acid-free paper
10 9 8 7 6 5 4 3 2 1

International Standard Book Number-10: 1-4398-0999-2 (Hardcover)
International Standard Book Number-13: 978-1-4398-0999-0 (Hardcover)

This book contains information obtained from authentic and highly regarded sources. Reprinted material is quoted with permission, and sources are indicated. A wide variety of references are listed. Reasonable efforts have been made to publish reliable data and information, but the author and the publisher cannot assume responsibility for the validity of all materials or for the consequence of their use.

No part of this book may be reprinted, reproduced, transmitted, or utilized in any form by any electronic, mechanical, or other means, now known or hereafter invented, including photocopying, microfilming, and recording, or in any information storage or retrieval system, without written permission from the publishers.

For permission to photocopy or use material electronically from this work, please access www.copyright.com (http://www.copyright.com/) or contact the Copyright Clearance Center, Inc. (CCC) 222 Rosewood Drive, Danvers, MA 01923, 978-750-8400. CCC is a not-for-profit organization that provides licenses and registration for a variety of users. For organizations that have been granted a photocopy license by the CCC, a separate system of payment has been arranged.

Trademark Notice: Product or corporate names may be trademarks or registered trademarks, and are used only for identification and explanation without intent to infringe.

Library of Congress Cataloging-in-Publication Data
Powell, Frank (Frank C. MD)
Rosacea : Diagnosis and Management / by Frank Powell.
p. ; cm.
Includes bibliographical references and index.
ISBN-13: 978-1-4200-7258-7 (hardcover : alk. paper)
ISBN-10: 1-4200-7258-7 (hardcover : alk. paper) 1. Rosacea. I. Title.
[DNLM: 1. Rosacea–therapy. 2. Rosacea–diagnosis. WR 430 P993 2008]
RL325.P69 2008
616.5'3–dc22
2008042775

For Corporate Sales and Reprint Permission call 212-520-2700 or write to: Sales Department, 52 Vanderbilt Avenue, 7th floor, New York, NY 10017.

**Visit the Informa Web site at
www.informa.com**

**and the Informa Healthcare Web site at
www.informahealthcare.com**

Preface

"Roses are red and so is my face
Pimples are sprouting all over the place..."
                    Robin Levine *(Red, White and Rosacea)*

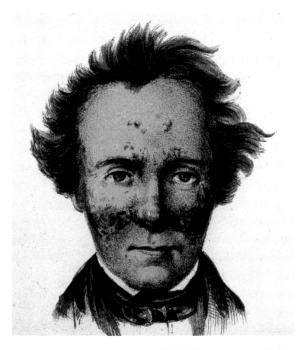

This 45 year old man has typical facial involvement with Rosacea. His physician from the 1800' recorded with surprise that he "never took liqueurs!!"

Shakespeare wrote about it, Rembrandt painted his self-portrait showing it, W.C. Fields made it his trademark in the movies, and both President Clinton and Princess Diana suffered from it!

Disorders that cause redness or inflammation of facial skin are a subject the general public has little knowledge of and about which the medical community has a poor understanding. At least one person in every ten in the adult population has a significant problem with increased facial redness (flushing, blushing, or rosacea), making these conditions more common than diabetes or asthma.

Disorders of frequent flushing or blushing may appear to be trivial complaints to those who do not suffer from them, but can be major problems to those afflicted, affecting both their personal and professional lives. Similarly, persistent redness and inflammation of the face or nose (rosacea) is often dismissed as a minor problem and sufferers can become the subject for "humorous" remarks. The enlargement or distortion of the nose (rhinophyma) that sometimes is seen in patients with rosacea is commonly (and incorrectly) thought to result from alcohol abuse, enhancing the social stigmatization that these individuals endure.

The reality is that people who develop these conditions have physical problems that arise for reasons that are not of their own making and that are not related to dietary or alcohol indiscretion. They suffer not only the discomfort of their disorders (which can affect not only the skin but the eyes as well), but at times social stigmatization.

This book is intended to bring a better level of knowledge of these problems to clinicians who treat patients with these disorders. It is hoped that it will stimulate interest as well as understanding so that the care of patients with rosacea will be improved.

Contents

Introduction

"She greeted me warmly, a little stoutish woman with keen eyes and a nose suspiciously red. . . ."

W Somerset Maugham (French Joe)

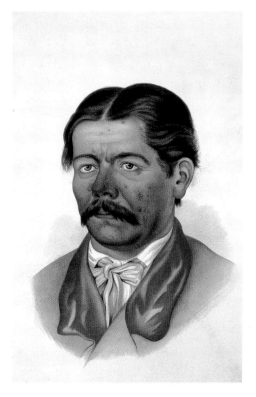

Figure 1 This beautifully illustrated figure shows an elegant middle aged gentleman of the nineteenth century with the clinical features of papulopustular rosacea (PPR). The erythema of the centrofacial region (nose, proximal cheeks and mid-forehead) and the papules and pustules are all well show.

BACKGROUND

Although rosacea is more common than diabetes and clearly visible to all, it is largely unknown to misunderstood by the general public. Knowledge relating to the epidemiology, etiology, and pathogenesis of this facial disorder that affects adults in middle age is limited. There are effective treatments of most of the manifestations of rosacea, but the mechanism of many treatments (particularly antibiotics) is unclear. In spite of this for the majority of patients a careful approach by their clinician to the diagnosis, classification, and management of their disorder will yield good results.

This illustrated work is intended to give clinicians an overview of the features of the different subtypes of rosacea, their differential diagnosis, and a practical approach to current therapeutic modalities. It is not intended to be an in-depth study of this disease. For a comprehensive text on acne and rosacea, readers are referred to the excellent work by Plewig and Kligman (1) and those readers who wish to review recent advances in knowledge will be best served by appropriate literature searches. The purpose of this work is to fill the gap that textbooks leave in the provision of solutions for individual patients with rosacea who often require their clinicians to be innovative in the approach to the management of their skin conditions. It is hoped that this will help those caring for patients with rosacea to diminish the impact of this unsightly and socially stigmatizing skin condition.

Traditional medical thinking about rosacea was often confused because the definition of the disease was vague. Several possibly unrelated conditions of facial redness were included under the broad title of "Rosacea." These ranged from patients with a propensity to frequent prolonged facial flushing being labelled as having "prerosacea," to patients who developed firm erythematous persistent facial papulonodules that demonstrated granulomas on histological examination being diagnosed as having "granulomatous rosacea."

The poor definition of rosacea was compounded by its assumed association with excessive consumption of alcohol. This deeply imbedded misconception in the minds of many members of the public has had the effect of stigmatizing patients with this disorder. The fact that the disorder is highly visible on the prominences of the face and difficult to mask cosmetically has made rosacea a skin condition that has a disproportionately large psychologic impact on sufferers.

Rosacea can negatively affect the patient's social and professional inter-actions. As a result, some patients feel insecure with low self-esteem and try to minimize social contacts, a situation that can lead to isolation and in extreme cases depression.

The frequency with which rosacea occurs in the general population is unclear but it probably affects at least 10% of individuals in middle age. A Swedish epidemiologic study of 809 office employees found a prevalence of 10% of rosacea (2). A recent epidemiologic study from Ireland (a country thought to have a high incidence of rosacea) of 1000 individuals found a prevalence of 13.9% of rosacea (3). The prevalence of rosacea probably depends on the genetic make-up of the population being studied. Most investigators agree that the condition is uncommon in dark-skinned individuals and occurs predominantly in those who are fair skinned and sun sensitive, particularly those of Celtic origin.

The etiology of rosacea is unknown. Because it occurs on sun-exposed skin in sun-sensitive patients, ultra violet light is thought to play a part in its pathogenesis. Some dermatologists suggest that facial vascular hyperreactivity is the underlying problem, while unusual bacteria or unusual behaviour of normal skin bacteria are suspected by others as being the cause. Another suggestion is that the overpopulation of demodex folliculorum mites seen in patients with rosacea, are important in its causation. It may well transpire that several of these factors are relevant and that each of the rosacea subtypes have different factors that are important to their initiation and pathogenesis. Further investigation of parameters such as facial blood flow, and follicular temperature, accurate measurements of degrees of erythema, the volume and consistency of the various constituents of sebum and meibomian gland secretion, accurate measurement of erythema and, skin pH etc., as well as study of the cutaneous microbiologic flora in rosacea is required to clarify its etiology and pathogenesis.

To understand rosacea, a working knowledge of the structure and function of normal skin is necessary. This work will begin with a review of the structure and function of human skin with particular reference to the face as the basis for the discussion of the clinical features and postulated pathogenic mechanisms of the different subtypes of rosacea.

Flushing and blushing are reactive vascular changes in the face seen in normal individuals. These take place in response to various stimuli, especially heat, certain foods, alcohol or emotional swings. Frequent and prolonged flushing can be a manifestation of abnormal psychosocial sensitivity or systemic illness such as the carcinoid syndrome. Frequent flushing can also be the presenting complaint of some patients with rosacea or accompany the inflammatory skin changes. The various types of flushing, their causation, and mechanism of action are reviewed in the next section together with the available treatments for this troublesome condition.

The basis for clinical diagnosis of rosacea and its classification into subsets is described in the next section. This classification provides a common language and has helped to clarify the various components of this disorder. This helps communication between researchers and physicians and ultimately will translate into better patient care. There are four subtypes of rosacea (4): Erythematotelang-iectatic rosacea (ETTR) is subtype 1, Papulopustular rosacea (PPR) is subtype 2, Phymatous rosacea (PR) is subtype 3 and Ocular rosacea (OR) is subtype 4. Each subtype is then graded according to disease severity (5). The grading system also assists clinicians in selecting therapy and in evaluating the patient's response to therapy.

In the following sections, each subtype of rosacea will be discussed with review of diagnostic criteria, distribution, clinical features, histology, differential diagnosis, and a guide to the appropriate treatment. Some patients may manifest more than one subset (for example patients with PPR may also have OR) and treatment of each subtype may need to be considered in the overall management of the patient.

Subtype 1 (ETTR) is probably the commonest subtype of rosacea. Its differentiation from facial photodamage can be problematic and may even be impossible in some patients, as the clinical features of both conditions overlap. Fortunately, the treatment for both these conditions is similar.

Subtype 2 (PPR) has a distinctive clinical presentation, and it was first described by dermatologists at the start of the 19th century. Some of these patients (typically males) may have in addition oily skin (usually individuals with rosacea have dry skin) and large inflammatory lesions difficult to distinguish from acne vulgaris. The treatment of Acne vulgaris and PPR is similar (with antibiotics or other agents) that again reduces the necessity for exact nosologic definitions. However, patients with rosacea are often poorly tolerant of the surface therapies used to treat acne vulagaris.

PR (subtype 3) is uncommon and usually occurs in older male patients. Rhinophyma is often thought of as being synonymous with end-stage rosacea but can occur in patients with mild rosacea or even in the absence of other features of rosacea in some individuals. Other phymatous changes are very rarely seen in patients with rosacea.

OR (subtype 4) is common and easily missed unless the clinician is aware of the association of rosacea and ocular inflammation and specifically enquires about its symptoms from the patient. It can be difficult or even impossible to diagnose OR in the absence of skin changes, as none of the clinical findings in the eye are exclusive to rosacea and there is no laboratory test that will confirm its diagnosis. Referral to an ophthalmologist is usually necessary for patients with persistent, moderate, or severe degrees of OR.

The principles of general skin care, the use of cosmetic cover, and the need for patient education regarding exacerbating "triggers" are important to the successful management of all patients with rosacea. These together with alternative and traditional approaches to the treatment of rosacea will be discussed in the last section of this work.

ACKNOWLEDGEMENT:

The older illustrations are included to illustrate the features of rosacea and similar facial skin conditions as well as individuals affected and to demonstrate the great detail that dermatologists of a former era paid to describing and illustrating this skin condition. They continue to provide valuable teaching tools for the physician of the present day.

The photographs shown here are of patients that have been under the care of the author. The impact of this disorder can be appreciated from the illustrations shown. I am grateful to these individuals for allowing their photographs to be taken and for the Photographic Department of the Mater Misericordiae University

Hospital for the superb quality of the images and for their unfailing assistance in the preparation of this work.

Dr Jonathan Wilkin's enthusiasm and depth of knowledge relating to rosacea has been a continued source of inspiration to me. He provided invaluable assistance in reviewing an early draft of this work and his encouraging and helpful comments and his contributions, particularly to the chapters on Flushing and General Considerations were all important.

Albert Kligman and Gerd Plewig are "maestros" of this disorder and are great sources of inspiration to the person interested in rosacea. I often "dip into" their works for renewed knowledge. As with many things that I have undertaken over the years this work would never have been completed without the help and encouragement of Maria.

REFERENCES

1. Plewig G and Kligman A. Acne Vulgaris and Rosacea. Springer-Verlag 2nd Edition 1993.
2. Berg M, Linden S. An epidemiological study of rosacea. Acta Derm Venereol 1989; 69:419–423.
3. McAleer MA, Fitzpatrick P, Powell FC. Prevalence and pathogenesis of Rosacea. Br J Dermatol 2008; 159(suppl 1):26.
4. Wilkin J, Dahl M, Detmar M, et al. Standard classification of rosacea: Report of the national rosacea society expert committee on the classification and staging of rosacea. J Am Acad Dermatol 2002; 46:584–587.
5. Wilkin J, Dahl M, Detmar M , et al. Standard grading system for rosacea: Report of the national rosacea society expert committee on the classification and staging of rosacea. J Am Acad Dermatol 2004; 50:907–912.

1

Structure, Function, Type, and Sensitivity of Skin

"Man must shed many skins
Before he attains
Even a measure of himself
And worldly things"
                    Von Goeth

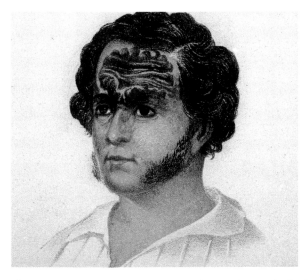

Figure 1 "Lichen agrius," a skin condition causing marked redness of the upper face, was first described in the 1800s and was thought to be due to continual heat exposure. The man shown here was a 45-year-old blacksmith who worked in a forge. Some dermatologists at that time thought that rosacea was caused by continual heat exposure. Lichen agrius is not listed as a skin disorder in modern textbooks and rosacea is no longer thought to be due to heat exposure.

To understand the clinical findings in rosacea, it is necessary to have an appreciation of the structure and function of normal facial skin. The skin is the outer living
layer that interacts with the environment. It is our protective barrier to potentially
harmful external biologic and physical agents and a retention barrier to prevent
loss of essential internal body fluids, electrolytes, proteins, and other substances.
It weighs between 4 and 5 kg and its total surface area is 1.5 m^2. It is a highly
complex continuously renewing organ comprising several distinctive sections that
merge with each other.

The functions of skin include immunologic competence and appreciation
of pain, temperature, touch, and pressure. It is intimately involved in body temperature regulation (especially the skin of the head and neck) and energy storage,
produces melanin pigment, (which is an effective screen protective against exposure to ultraviolet light), excretes water and salt, and manufactures vitamin D.
Besides these important physiologic functions, the skin of the face in particular has considerable psychosocial and aesthetic importance. People often use the
phrase that they took an individual at "face value," and some emotions may be
displayed not only by facial expression but also by altering facial blood flow (e.g.
shame, embarrassment, fear) (Fig. 2).

SKIN STRUCTURE

Human skin consists of three distinctive but integrated sections: the *epidermis*,
dermis, and *subcutaneous fat* (Fig. 3). The epidermis is the outermost section
of the skin, forming the avascular but biologically active skin surface. Cells
proliferate in the deepest layer of the epidermis (the actively dividing basal
layer) and move upward to the surface corneal layer. Cells in the basal layer
have an "upright" or "columnar" orientation, as they appear to "stand" on the
basement membrane that forms the junction between the epidermis and the
layer deeper to it (the dermis). As the cells migrate upward in the epidermis
from the basal layer to form the squamous layer, their cell walls become stiffer,
their constituents change, and the cells flatten. The internal structures of the
squamous cells appear to degenerate as they move further upward to become the
granular layer. By the time the cells of the granular layer reach the epidermal
surface they have lost their nucleus and become corneal cells (corneocytes)
forming the outer protective keratin sheet called the "horny layer"—the most
important barrier layer of the epidermis. The progressive differentiation process
by which basal cells biochemically and morphologically transform into the cells
of the horny layer is called keratinization (Fig. 4). In time, the cells of the
horny layer are desquamated into the surface film and subsequently lost to the
environment.

The **surface film** is a hydrolipidic emulsion formed by the secretions from
skin glands (sebaceous, eccrine, and apocrine) containing shed cells, occasional
yeast and bacterial organisms, and on the face, occasional demodex folliculorum
mites. The functions of this surface film are not known, but it may contribute to

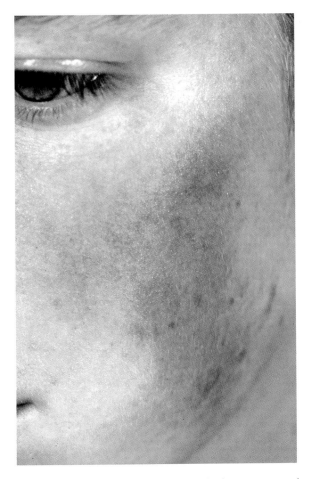

Figure 2 Blotchy erythema on the cheek of a young man who is flushing with embarrassment and self-consciousness.

skin integrity by providing a protective lubricant to its surface strengthening the barrier function of the stratum corneum. The quality or composition of the skin surface film may vary in different individuals, possibly depending on their skin type (see later). Its integrity is also probably influenced by environmental factors such as exposure to wind and ultraviolet light, relative humidity, air conditioning, and atmospheric pollutants. All topical products and medications interact with this film. Agents that peel or "exfoliate" the skin as well as vigorously cleansing and some alcohol-containing or perfumed cosmetic agents are likely to change the nature of the skin surface film. Such agents often increase skin sensitivity and are usually poorly tolerated by rosacea patients.

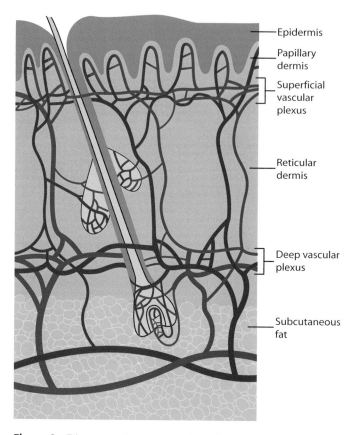

Epidermis

Papillary
dermis

Superficial
vascular
plexus

Reticular
dermis

Deep vascular
plexus

Subcutaneous
fat

Figure 3 Diagrammatic representation of a cross-section of human skin showing the epidermis, dermis, subcutaneous fat and related structures. Note the prominent hair follicle with a large terminal hair and relatively small sebaceous glands at either side. The superficial and deep vascular networks are clearly seen.

Practice Point: A 35-year-old lady was prescribed 10% benzoyl peroxide for "acne vulgaris." Within 3 days, she developed facial soreness, redness, and peeling and sought another medical opinion. Clinical examination showed the correct diagnosis to be rosacea. She was prescribed 1% hydrocortisone cream to be applied twice daily to her face for a week and doxycycline 100 mg daily. The benzoyl peroxide was stopped. The soreness and peeling settled rapidly.

Comment: Unlike patients with acne vulgaris, patients with rosacea rarely tolerate topical peeling or drying medications. Mild topical steroids can be safely used for a short period to treat irritant reactions of facial skin in rosacea patients.

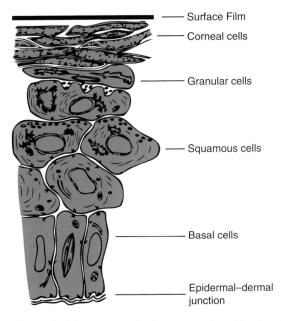

Surface Film

Corneal cells

Granular cells

Squamous cells

Basal cells

Epidermal–dermal junction

Figure 4 Keratinization is the process by which basal cells are transformed into the corneocytes of the horny layer. This figure is a diagrammatic representation of the epidermis showing the surface film, horny, granular, squamous, and basal layers. The basal cells "sit" on the epidermal–dermal junction, which separates the epidermis from the dermis.

Patients with rosacea often complain of increased facial skin sensitivity and a sensation of "stinging" when exposed to minor stimuli such as wind, temperature change, and perfumated products. Their abnormal skin sensitivity can be demonstrated by the lactic acid skin test.

The surface film sits on the **horny layer**, which is the outermost cellular layer of the epidermis. It comprises a tightly formed network of keratinized cells (corneocytes) stacked one upon the other, cemented together by intercellular lipids with intercellular bridges called corneodesmosomes that combine to give a "brick wall" appearance to this layer (Fig. 5). This structure forms a formidable outer barrier for the skin. Corneocytes are the end product of keratinization initiated in the basal layer of the epidermis. Although lacking a nucleus and technically "dead," they play a vital role in the body's defence system and the integrity of the skin. Exposed to continual environmental interaction, this waterproof, flexible, almost impenetrable barrier depends on both its intercellular lipids and the hydrolipidic film on the skin surface for its functionality (1). The cells on the surface of the horny layer are eventually shed into the surface film consequent to biochemical alteration to the intercellular lipid-rich cement. The horny layer has the ability to adapt to the body's needs and function by varying its thickness and protective capability. On skin areas exposed to frequent friction such as the palms of the

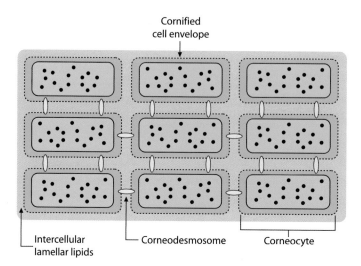

Cornified
cell envelope

Intercellular
lamellar lipids

Corneodesmosome

Corneocyte

Figure 5 The horny layer of the skin is said to resemble a "brick wall" structure, the corneocytes stacked one upon the other with intercellular lipids and interconnecting corneodesmosomes contributing to provide a substantial protective barrier for the skin.

hands and the soles of the feet, the horny layer can be four to five times thicker than it is on the face where frictional forces are minimal.

"He who has thick skin takes no notice of a flea bite."
Old proverb

The horny layer also thickens in response to repeated ultraviolet light exposure and contains UV-blocking melanin particles manufactured by the pigment-producing melanocytes of the basal layer and transferred from them through their dendritic processes to the upward-migrating squamous cells. The horny layer is the primary cutaneous defence system against biologic agents such as bacteria, yeasts, and fungi as well as a physical protection against the various environmental agents that come into contact with skin on a daily basis. The horny layer is also important in homeostasis by preventing loss of water, body fluids, and electrolytes through the skin. A defect of the horny layer, as happens with superficial abrasions or burns, leaves the skin open to infection and loss of serum. With extensive deficiency of the horny layer, the loss of fluids and electrolytes may be so severe as to threaten the integrity of the person affected.

The **granular layer** that lies under the horny layer is composed of diamond-shaped cells derived from the underlying squamous layer. The cells of this layer show signs of degeneration and shed their nucleus as they move upward to form the horny layer. The prominent cytoplasmic granules (from which the layer derives its name) are amorphous protein particles called profilaggrin that transform into filaggrin and help to cement together the cells of the horny layer.

The **squamous layer** composed of partially flattened cells lies directly beneath the granular layer, and keratin and soluble proteins such as involucrin (an integral component of the barrier quality of the horny layer) are produced here.

The **basal layer** is the proliferative or germinative layer from which the other layers of the epidermis arise. It has been calculated that the time taken for cells to move from the basal layer to the skin surface (the epidermal turnover time) is approximately 30 days, a period that varies with age, season, pregnancy, and skin disease. The epidermal turnover time in patients with rosacea appears to be normal.

Thus, the epidermis is an integrated, dynamic, biologically active outer skin layer that provides protection to the body through the process of keratinization. It is continually being shed and regenerated. An indication of the extent of this process is the fact that it has been estimated that several million cells are shed everyday from the skin surface of the average person.

The epidermis also contains specialized cells. Approximately 1 of every 10 cells in the basal layer is a **melanocyte**, which produces melanin pigment in specialized organelles (melanosomes). The colour of skin (black, brown, white) is determined by the degree of melanization of these melanosomes; the more heavily melanized the melanosomes, the darker the skin colour. Melanocytes manufacture the "pigment umbrella" for the skin, each one transferring melanosomes to several squamous cells which carry these in their upward migration to the horny layer maximising the UV screening effect. Patients who have skin that is poorly melanized make up the majority of rosacea sufferers. Sun damage (solar elastosis) is commonly seen in the upper dermis of skin biopsies taken from the face of patients with rosacea reflecting their susceptibility to solar radiation.

Ultraviolet light can also be beneficial to the skin as it stimulates the production of biologically important vitamin D in epidermal keratinocytes. The epidemic of rickets (a bone disease due to a deficiency of vitamin D) in the 1800s in London occurred when children from the deprived sections of that city had minimal UV exposure (due to poor housing conditions) combined with a diet deficient in vitamin D.

Langerhans cells are immunologically competent cells of the epidermis found scattered just above the basal cells. These cells were first described by Paul Langerhans in 1868 when he was still a medical student, but their function remained unknown until fairly recently. They have long "dendritic" processes that form an extensive branching network in the suprabasal epidermis (Fig. 6). The purpose of this dendritic network of immune competent cells appears to be the trapping, processing, and the presentation of antigens to lymphocytes migrating from the dermal blood vessels. Langerhans cells "orchestrate" the complex cutaneous immune response to foreign matter. They also have an important role in cutaneous cancer surveillance. They are depleted by ultraviolet light and this possibly contributes to the susceptibility of skin malignancies developing in patients who have a lot of sun exposure.

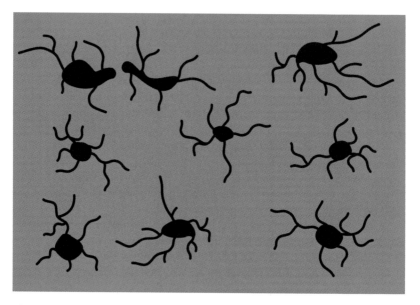

Figure 6 Diagrammatic representation of the type of dendritic meshwork formed in the epidermis by the bone marrow–derived Langerhan cells. These provide a comprehensive network of immune surveillance cells.

KEY POINTS

- Several million epidermal cells are shed every day.
- With increasing age, the rate of skin shedding slows and skin roughens.
- The normal rate of epidermal turnover is approximately 30 days.
- The rate of epidermal turnover varies according to season (faster in summer) and during pregnancy.
- A skin surface film of lipid secretions, dead cells, and organisms covers the stratum corneum.
- The stratum corneum is the key barrier layer of the skin and varies in thickness according to site.
- Melanocytes manufacture melanin in melanosomes to protect against ultra-violet exposure.
- The degree of melanization of melanosomes determines skin colour and sensitivity to sunburn.
- Melanosomes form a cutaneous ultraviolet protective "pigment umbrella."
- Langerhans cells orchestrate the skin's immune response by antigen pre-sentation to lymphocytes.
- Vitamin D is manufactured in the epidermis by keratinocytes when exposed to ultraviolet light.

The **dermis** comprises the middle section of the skin. Its thickness varies, being relatively thin on the face and thicker on the back. The dermis has been referred to as the "under felt of the epidermal carpet" and is separated from the epidermis by the basement membrane zone. Multiple tiny fibrils and filaments pass through this zone to anchor the epidermis to the dermis. The basement membrane zone provides mechanical support for the overlying basal cells and is a semipermeable filter through which nutrients and cells pass via the rich vascular network of the dermis to the epidermis. The dermis provides the structural support to the skin. It is composed of a matrix of **collagen**—a multistranded interwoven threadlike material that packs and strengthens the middle layer of the skin surrounding and supporting the blood vessels, nerves, and lymphatics. Solar Elastosis is the term used for collagen degenerated by exposure to ultraviolet light. As already mentioned it is a consistent histological finding in the skin of patients with rosacea. Collagen fibers develop cross-linkages with aging and collagenase enzymes (which are activated by ultraviolet light) metabolize the fibrous structure. Collagen is constantly being replenished by cells in the dermis called fibroblasts. **Elastic fibers** constitute only 2% of the dermis, but confer the important stretching quality to the skin, while **ground substance** is an amorphous material that fills the spaces between the fibrillar and cellular components of the dermis giving it a resilient and turgid quality.

The dermis is also the location of the oil-producing sebaceous glands, the sweat-producing eccrine glands, and the hair follicles. These latter structures are classified as being terminal, vellus, or sebaceous depending on the type of hair produced in the follicle.

The follicles of the central face, the area typically affected by rosacea, produce tiny hairs and have large related sebaceous glands. They are classified as "sebaceous follicles."

The sebaceous glands of the face are richly vascularized, androgen-sensitive glands that secrete an oily emulsion called **sebum**. This is composed of cholesterol, cholesterol esters, triglycerides, wax esters, squalene, and fatty acids. Sebum passes via the follicular canal to the skin surface and provides the protective and lubricating oil for the surface film of the face. Man has more sebaceous glands than any other known animal. These glands are largest and most active on the so-called "T zone" of the face (central forehead, nose, and central chin) and are central to the pathogenesis of acne vulgaris. Their relevance to the production of the inflammatory lesions of rosacea is hotly debated.

Skin temperature affects the viscosity of sebum and also its ability to spread on the skin surface. It has been suggested that the temperature of the skin of the face in patients with rosacea is higher than normal, which could affect the viscosity of sebum altering its lubricating qualities and possibly increasing skin sensitivity. Surprisingly, studies of the temperature of the skin in rosacea patients have shown conflicting results and this fundamental piece of information remains to be confirmed.

In addition to sebum, the follicular canals of the facial skin contains a melange of cell detritus, flakes of keratinized cells, and **microorganisms** such as

Corynebacterium acnes and *Pityrosporum ovale* as well as *Demodex folliculorum* mites. *D. folliculorum* mites are greatly increased in number in the facial skin of patients with rosacea and may be of pathogenic importance (2).

Meibomian glands are modified sebaceous glands, which are found in the upper and lower tarsal plates of the eyelids. Their openings are seen as tiny pores behind the eyelashes (cilia). The function of the meibomian glands is to produce the oil component of tear secretions, which is an aqueous/lipid mixture. The meibum secreted by these glands is rich in wax and sterol esters and contains triglycerides and free fatty acids. The tear film has important antimicrobial as well as lubricant properties. The functioning of these glands are often adversely affected in patients who have ocular rosacea leading to abnormally rapid tear breakup time and causing a sensation of "dry eyes."

Practice Point: A 55-year-old man was prescribed isotretinoin 1.5 mgs/kg for early rhinophyma. He rapidly developed soreness of his eyes, which progressively deteriorated. Secondary infected blepharitis followed and required treatment with topical and systemic antibiotics (and discontinuation of isotretinoin). Artificial tear replacement was necessary.

   Comment: Isotretinoin may further compromise meibomian gland dysfunction in rosacea patients leading to profound ocular dryness and susceptibility to secondary bacterial infection. It should be used with caution and in low dosages only in these patients.

There are two main horizontal **vascular plexuses** in the skin (superficial and deep) with multiple intercommunicating vessels and together they form a vast network of reactive blood vessels (Fig. 3). Alteration of the calibre of these vessels plays an important role in temperature regulation and homeostasis. Under thermal stress conditions, vasodilatation can increase skin blood flow up to 10-fold. This allows body heat to be lost rapidly through the skin because heat conductivity of blood is high and convection and radiation of heat from the skin occurs quickly. Discharge of sweat from the eccrine glands and its subsequent evaporation from the skin surface also helps to reduce body temperature. Thermoreceptor nerve endings in the skin play an important role in the monitoring of skin temperature and, together with the multiple thermostats in the central nervous system, function to coordinate the regulation of core temperature. The skin of the face has an abundance of blood vessels, even though it requires and consumes little oxygen. Some investigators feel that the basis of flushing in patients with rosacea lies in an abnormal reactivity of these vessels, vasodilatating for prolonged periods in response to stimuli such as minor temperature change, emotion or ingestion of agents such as alcohol, hot beverages, or spicy foods.

Lymphatics are small blind-ended afferent capillaries lined by a single layer of epithelium, which run parallel to the vascular network outlined above. The smallest lymphatic vessels begin in the upper dermis and drain lymphatic fluid from this region, emptying into a superficial plexus, which in turn flows through interconnecting vessels into deeper plexuses located between the dermis and the subcutaneous fat, and thence onward to the central lymphatic system. The facial swelling seen in patients with some forms of edematous rosacea (Morbihan disease) is thought to be related to malfunction of the lymph-draining network of the face. Facial massage in a rotatory fashion to increase lymphatic drainage has been promoted as a treatment for this type of edematous rosacea.

The skin of the face is richly **innervated**. The nerve endings in the skin form the "terminus" of the peripheral nervous system. Free nerve endings are also present in the eyelids and form a complex around hair follicles.

Motor innervation to the skin may result in increased sweating, vasoconstriction, or erector pili muscles contraction causing "goose pimples."

Some rosacea researchers feel that neurovascular peptide release from cutaneous nerve endings may be important in the causation of rosacea.

KEY POINTS

- The dermis is the middle layer of the skin separated from the epidermis by the dermoepidermal junction.
- The thickness of the dermis varies according to the site (thick on the back and thin on the face).
- Collagen makes up the majority of the substance of the dermis and is arranged in intertwining fibers.
- Collagen fibers are manufactured by fibroblasts in the dermis.
- Elastic fibers and ground substance make up the minority of the dermis.
- The dermis contains a rich network of blood vessels arranged in horizontal tracks.
- Lymphatic vessels run parallel to blood vessels in the dermis.
- The sebaceous glands of the skin and the pilosebaceous follicles are found in the dermis.
- Meibomian glands of the eyelid are modified sebaceous glands.
- Eccrine (sweat) and apocrine glands are in the deep dermis where it merges with the subcutaneous fat.
- Nerve fibers and free nerve endings can be identified in the dermis.
- The subcutaneous fat lies beneath the dermis and serves as an energy store, insulation, and protective cushion to the skin.

The **subcutaneous fat** is the deepest layer of the skin and sits on top of fascia, muscle, or bone. It is usually not marked in the face. Subcutaneous fat is "the cushioning layer" or "shock absorber" of the skin and provides padded insulation to conserve heat. It is also a major energy store for the skin. Larger blood vessels, nerves, lymphatics, as well as some of the sweat glands are found in the subcutaneous fat.

Table 1 Summary of Skin Functions

Protection	Horny layer/surface film/Langerhans cells/melanocytes/nerves/ subcutaneous fat
Heat regulation	Dermal blood vessels/eccrine secretions/subcutaneous fat
Sensation	Free nerve endings
Absorption	Transepidermal into dermal blood vessels/lymphatics
Excretion	Eccrine/apocrine/sebaceous glands/possible excretion of "toxins"
Synthesis	Keratin/vitamin D after sun exposure
Attraction	Turgidity and "youthful" appearance/cultural skin colour preferences
Communication	Emotional changes manifested in facial skin/electrical changes (lie detector)

SKIN FUNCTION

Many of the functions of the skin have already been referred to during the description of the skin structure (Table 1). In addition to those already described, the absorptive quality of the skin is increasingly being used as a means of transcutaneous delivery of medications to avoid their potential irritating effect on the lining of the stomach.

Excretion (of water and sodium chloride and probably other materials) takes place through the skin, but there has been little research focused on this aspect of skin function to date. Some naturopathic physicians and nutritionists believe that cutaneous elimination of "toxins" is an important skin function. They suggest that defective cutaneous excretion of toxic substances can lead to the inflammatory changes in the skin of patients with both acne vulgaris and rosacea. As already indicated vitamin D synthesis takes place in the skin. Activated vitamin D has recently been shown to have a role in the regulation of antimicrobial peptides (AMPs) and may be significant in the pathogenesis of rosacea as it appears that some such peptides (cathelicidins) are abnormally processed and may lead to inflammation in the skin.

Young, wrinkle-free, healthy, smooth, blemish-free skin is attractive and physical attraction is an important skin function. The cosmetic industry makes billions of dollars in profits from their products, which they claim make the skin appear more attractive.

Skin also provides a means of communication, as emotional changes can be signaled by blushing, going pale, or sweating. The tendency for rosacea sufferers to flush readily thus sends inappropriate signals to people they interact with.

Patients with rosacea are often acutely aware that their skin appears unattractive, a fact that physicians caring for these patients should not overlook or minimize.

SKIN TYPE

The level of reactivity of an individual's skin when exposed to sunlight is often referred to as their "skin type." Individuals with pale, sun-sensitive skin that always burns and never tans when exposed to sunlight are said to have type 1

Table 2 The Different Skin Types (Fitzpatrick)

Type 1	White skin/always burn, never tan/freckle on sun exposure/red/blond hair, blue/grey eyes
Type 2	White skin/burn initially, eventually form poor tan/freckle, etc., as type 1
Type 3	Sallow skin/tan easily but can burn/black/brown hair, brown eyes
Type 4	Brown skin, does not easily burn/hair + eyes as above
Type 5	Asian skin/rarely burn /brown eyes/dark hair
Type 6	African black skin/brown eyes, dark hair, hardly ever burn

skin. Those people with pale skin that usually burns with exposure to sunlight, but may eventually develops a poor tan are said to have type 2 skin. Persons with skin types 1 and 2 have skin that freckles readily. Individuals with sallow skin that rarely burns when exposed to sunlight and readily develops a tan are said to have type 3 skin. Individuals with type 4 skin have skin of a deep sallow to light brown colour that hardly ever burns when exposed to sunlight but rather tans and darkens readily. People of Asian origin are said to have type 5 skin while individuals with black skin are regarded as having type 6 skin.

Hair and eye color also may be related to the tendency to burn in the sun. Those individuals with sun-sensitive easily burnt skin (skin types 1 and 2) often have fair light brown or reddish hair and blue, green, or gray eyes, while those who tan readily (skin type 3 and 4) and those with skin types 5 and 6 usually have dark brown or black hair and brown eyes (see Table 2).

Studies of patients with rosacea have consistently shown that the majority of individuals who develop this disorder have skin types 1 or 2. This, and the fact that rosacea occurs on the facial prominences as well as its appearance on the scalp of male patients when this is exposed by alopecia, suggests that sunlight is involved in the pathogenesis of the disease.

SKIN SENSITIVITY

Patients with rosacea often complain of increased facial skin "sensitivity," most frequently during the summer months when additional ultraviolet exposure may be a factor (3). This is usually manifested as redness and a stinging, burning, or itchy sensation of the skin.

The cause of sensitive skin is not fully understood. An impaired skin barrier function with an increase in transepidermal water loss is a common feature and has been mentioned earlier. Skin hydration depends on moisture diffusion to the horny layer and fluid secreted by sweat glands. The rate of evaporation of moisture from the skin surface in part reflects the moisture-retaining ability of the horny layer and surface film and its lipid content. An imbalance of one or several of these elements in patients with rosacea may predispose them to having "sensitive skin." Skin sensitivity is evaluated by the "lactic acid test" which scores the intensity of the sensation of stinging induced by the application of a 5% solution of lactic acid to the skin surface.

KEY POINTS

- Skin has many important biological functions.
- Facial vasculature has a thermoregulatory role.
- Facial flushing in rosacea patients conveys inappropriate social signals to others.
- Most individuals with rosacea have sun sensitive types 1 or 2 skin.
- Patients with rosacea have sensitive, easily irritated skin.
- Contact allergy should be considered in a patient with rosacea with unexplained skin deterioration in spite of appropriate therapy.

Although rarely sensitized by the topical antibiotics used to treat facial rosacea, patients with rosacea may develop an allergic contact dermatitis to preservatives, perfumes or other agents contained in topical cosmetic products, or to the topical antibiotics used to treat ocular infections. Unexplained deterioration of rosacea in spite of appropriate therapy may indicate the necessity for patch testing in such patients.

Individuals with sensitive skin (including those with rosacea) react vigorously to stimuli that persons with normal skin do not (e.g., ultraviolet radiation, wind, and temperature change) and their increased sensitivity can be shown by the lactic acid test.

REFERENCES

1. Pons-Guiraud A. Dry skin in dermatology: A complex physiopathology. JEADV 2007; 21(suppl 2):1–4.
2. Bonner E, Eustace P, Powell FC. The demodex mite population in Rosacea. J Am Acad Dermatol 1993; 28:443–448.
3. Guzman-Sanchez DA, Ishiuji Y, Patel T, et al. Enhanced skin blood flow and sensitivity to noxious heat stimuli in papulopustular rosacea. J Am Acad Dermatol 2007; 57:800–805.

FURTHER READING

Cork MJ. The importance of skin barrier function. J Dermatol Treatment 1997; 8:s7–s13.
Comment: This is an excellent account of skin barrier function that focuses on the disorder atopic dermatitis. Many of the same principles apply to patients with rosacea.
Fitzpatrick TB. The validity and practicality of sun-reactive skin types 1 through 6. Arch Dermatol 1998; 124: 869.
Comment: The Fitzpatrick skin types are fundamental to categorizing the reactivity of skin to ultraviolet light and may also be helpful in predicting skin sensitivity.

2

Flushing and Blushing

"Her pure and eloquent blood
Spoke in her cheeks,
And so distinctly wrought
That one might almost say
Her body thought. . . ."
  Spenser, *The Faerie Queen*

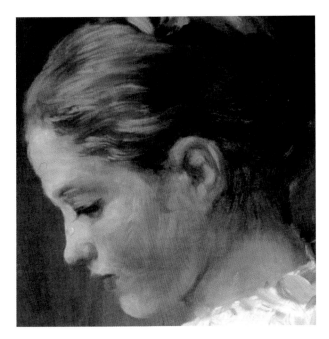

Figure 1 This portrait of young girl shows her slightly flushed cheek as an attractive feature. Note also the blotchy nature of the flush on her cheek and its extension up to her ear.

Although frequent flushing or blushing are not necessarily a component of the clinical picture in all patients with rosacea, they are present sufficiently often enough to merit review here, and are the first features of rosacea to appear in some patients.

DEFINITION

The words flushing and blushing are often used interchangeably but in fact these terms should more correctly be used to designate different conditions which may have disparate initiating factors.

Flushing is an unpleasant sudden intense diffuse reddening of the face (and often other areas such as the neck and chest), which is an exaggeration of the normal vasodilatatory response to hyperthermia or other factors. It is caused by a precipitous extensive facial vasodilatation leading to increased cutaneous blood flow. Flushing may be precipitated by dietary factors, alcohol or other drugs, environmental temperature change, hormonal change, rarely systemic disease, or may occur for no apparent reason. Both men and women are equally susceptible to flushing. No particular age group is more vulnerable than another, but menopausal women are particularly affected because of hormonal changes. Flushing may be accompanied by sweating and occasionally symptoms such as wheezing, diarrhea, or headache. The facial redness persists 5 minutes or longer in most individuals. After the flush resolves some individuals may have a feeling of weakness or tiredness.

Blushing implies an episodic, sudden, transient, often blotchy, involuntary reddening of the face (and often the sides of the neck, and ears), which is precipitated by emotion or psychologic upset (shame, anger, embarrassment, guilt, pleasure, or anxiety). It has been suggested that displaying moral emotions via flushing serves important psychologic functions, but in some sensitive individuals, the mildest of emotions may trigger flushing, which may inhibit their normal social interactions.

Darwin said that blushing was "the most peculiar and the most human of all expressions" and he was convinced that no animal actually blushed. On hearing Darwin's views Mark Twain apparently retorted that "Humans are the only animals that blush, or that need to!

> *"Gabriel coloured as if he felt he had made a mistake . . .*
> *The high colour of his cheeks pushed upwards even to his forehead*
> *Where it scattered itself in a few formless patches of pale red . . ."*
> James Joyce, *The Dead*

Blushing is involuntary and cannot easily be inhibited by mental effort. Awareness of the tendency of blushing to occur in certain social situations can cause a susceptible person to develop a type of anticipatory anxiety, which increases the likelihood that blushing will in fact occur. If this anxiety becomes persistent, it can lead to social phobia with such individuals developing a psychologic fear of situations in which they are likely to blush. The term "ery-throphobia" or "morbidly shy" is sometimes applied to this almost pathologic fear of blushing. Blushing is more common in younger individuals and the tendency often diminishes in later adolescence. Young girls appear to be most susceptible to blushing and it is often considered an attractive feature in this group. Blushing is not usually accompanied by facial sweating or other systemic symptoms but there is often a mild tingling or burning sensation in the areas of skin affected by the blush. Blushing usually causes a transient facial redness that lasts less than 5 minutes and there is no residual feeling of weakness or tiredness afterward.

The social interpretation of frequent blushing has changed over the years. In Victorian England, an inability to blush was considered an "outward sign of inner failings, most especially, moral weakness and lack of conscience." Excessive blushing, on the other hand, was said to suggest "evidence of inner moral derange-ment and often betrayed the chronic masturbator." While major social changes have taken place since those times, the tendency to blush may still be misinter-preted as a sign of lying or insecurity and in men as an indication of homosexuality. These factors increase the disease burden for patients with rosacea.

When both flushing and blushing resolve, they leave the skin looking com-pletely normal. It can be difficult to distinguish between flushing and blushing, and there are patients in whom there is a mixed clinical picture making accurate classification impossible and the terms will be used interchangeably henceforth in this book.

Flushing and blushing occurs with equal frequency in persons with skin of colour but can be difficult to discern clinically, being recognised primarily by relative or close friend.

DISTRIBUTION

While it is recognized that there is a crossover in the distribution of flushing and blushing, flushing is usually more widespread; often extending in a diffuse fashion from the hair-line (sometimes even spreading to the scalp) to involve the neck and the upper anterior chest. A blotchy flush that is sometimes seen in female subjects which is localized to the neck and upper anterior chest and which occurs in the absence of facial flushing has been referred to as the "Flush of Venus". Occasion-ally, (especially if associated with systemic disease), flushing can be generalized. Rarely, both flushing and blushing may be seen in the epigastric region (1).

Blushing is usually limited to the lateral cheeks and is often blotchy in appearance (Figs. 2 and 3). Occasionally, the ears redden with blushing and the sides of the neck may be involved.

> *"Suddenly a thought came like a full blown rose,*
> *Flushing his brow, and in his pained heart*
> *Made purple riot."*
> John Keats, *The Eve of St. Agnes*

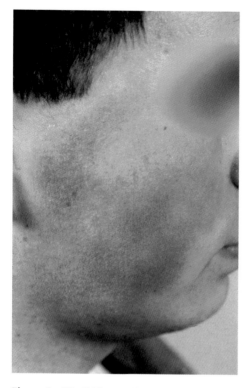

Figure 2   The "skip areas" of pallor on the upper lateral cheek are prominent in this young man with frequent blushing which caused social inhibition. Note how the area of blush extends to the preauricular area. His ears also reddened with blushing.

Practice Point: The teenaged boy in Figure 2 began to avoid attending school because of his tendency to flush bright red when attention was focused on him in class. This caused him intense anxiety and he desperately wanted to avoid the situations in which he was likely to blush. His mother thought that he would develop rosacea and was worried that he would develop rhinophyma. Both he and his mother had viewed pictures of rosacea and rhinophyma on the internet and were very concerned.

   Comment: Frequent flushing and anxiety often go hand in hand in this age group. Rosacea is rarely consequent to this type of problem. Reassurance and counseling (sometimes for both the patient and the parent!) are often helpful and systemic medications should be restricted to cases where flushing is having a major impact on the persons ability to function socially. Low dose beta blockers (e.g. propranolol 10–20 mgs daily) can be helpful in diminishing both the tendency to flush and the associated anxiety. Rhinophyma is not a likely outcome in this young man.

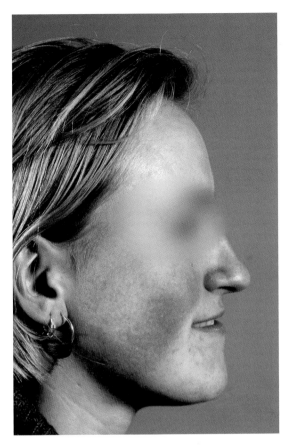

Figure 3 This figure shows another young patient who complained of frequent and prolonged blushing. Note the involvement of the lateral cheeks with islands of pallor within the reddened skin and the redness of the ears.

BACKGROUND

As we have already noted Charles Darwin was one of the first people to study flushing and blushing. In his book, *The expressions of the Emotions in Man and Animals* published in 1872, he described the progressive evolution of a flush up the sides of the neck to the cheeks and forehead (2). He suggested an association between a "nervous predisposition" and flushing, and pointed out that individuals who flushed frequently were "psychologically vulnerable." He noted that animals (apart from monkeys) did not flush and none blushed which he related to their lack of emotional sensibility. Following Darwin's famous publication the association between facial reddening and emotions became firmly embedded in the public psyche. This has lead inadvertently to some curious theories relating to the etiology of rosacea.

The possible association of flushing (or blushing) to the development of rosacea has been debated for many years.

Some investigators have even suggested that individuals who have sensitive facial skin and flush frequently should be classified as having "pre-rosacea", but the evidence to support this is lacking.

The validity of the results of retrospective studies of the frequency of flushing in patients with rosacea must be open to question because of the lack of clear definition of both rosacea and the type of facial reaction that constituted facial flushing or blushing. It is generally accepted that some patients with rosacea, in particular those who have erythematotelangiectatic (subtype 1) rosacea, appear to have labile facial vasculature and are likely to flush when exposed to a warm environment or with certain dietary stimulants. Some of these individuals may recall a tendency to redden easily from childhood, and state that they blushed more readily than their contemporaries when they were younger. Some may even recall a familial tendency to flushing. This suggests that there is a subset of individuals who have facial blood vessels that are constitutionally hyperreactive manifested by a tendency to blush easily in childhood. Some of these people may later develop the persistent facial erythema and telangiectasias of erythematotelangiectatic rosacea (ETTR), but this outcome is by no means inevitable and prospective studies of large numbers of patients are needed to answer this important question. The development of ETTR in these patients may in fact be consequent to exposure of their reactive facial skin to the irritating effects of temperature, wind, and ultraviolet light rather than the effects of frequent flushing.

The significance of flushing to the pathogenesis of other subtypes of rosacea, especially papulopustular rosacea (PPR) subtype 2, is unclear. Patients who have subtype 2 rosacea often do not have a history of flushing readily. Some of these patients who do flush have become very self-conscious about their facial skin condition and blush when attention is drawn to their rosacea. Similarly, their inflamed skin may redden additionally on exposure to heat but these are probably secondary effects. Flushing is not a frequent accompaniment of rhinophyma, and sometimes, but not frequently, is seen in our patients with ocular rosacea.

CLINICAL FEATURES

An interesting clinical feature of the distribution of the erythema in patients who blush is the presence of "skip areas" or "islands of sparing" where the skin remains pale (Figs. 2 and 3). The cause of this is unclear, but it may reflect areas of the face in which the dermal blood vessels different or are less reactive to the vasodilatatory stimulus.

The presence or absence of accompanying sweating with flushing can be a useful clinical feature. It's presence (sweating) implies involvement of the autonomic nervous system in the mechanism of the flush.

From a clinical perspective, flushing can be conveniently divided into two major categories, wet or dry flushes. If there is an associated sweating (*wet flushes*), this usually implies involvement of the autonomic nervous system in the genesis

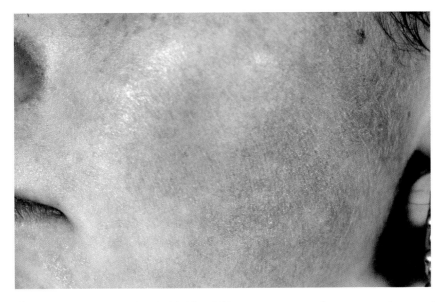

Figure 4 The flushed shiny facial skin of this woman suggests the menopausal cause of her flushing. Typically accompanied by sweating (hot or "wet" flushing) the menopause is one of the commonest causes of flushing in middle aged female patients.

of the flush. This type of flushing is more likely to result from a rise in the environmental temperature, the ingestion of hot food or hot drinks, or vigorous exercise. A counter effect to these stimulants can be produced by lowering the ambient temperature (by the use of air conditioning, for example); the ingestion of cold liquids; or the retention of ice chips in the mouth ("ice chip therapy"); as well as wearing of loose light clothing.

Menopausal flushing is usually diffuse on the face and the skin often appears shiny (Fig. 4) as typically this type of flushing is associated with sweating (so called "hot flushes"). The average hot flush lasts about 4 minutes, but can last from several seconds to 10 minutes. Their frequency ranges from several per week to hourly. Women who are underweight, those who do little exercise, and smokers appear to be at increased risk (3). It would appear that women with hot flushes have an increased body core temperature and a reduced thermoneutral zone (a zone between shivering and sweating) (4). Therefore, a relatively mild stimulus will give rise to cutaneous vasodilatation in these individuals. Effective treatments for hot flushes should restore the normal thermoneutral zone, but studies of medications used to treat menopausal flushing are hampered by the high rate of placebo effect (up to 30% of individuals respond to placebo agents in some studies). Hormonal therapy (HRT) is the standard treatment and can decrease the frequency and severity of hot flushes by up to 90%. However, long-term estrogen therapy is associated with an increased risk of heart and thromboembolic disease as well as possibly increasing the susceptibility of the individual to the development of breast cancer and so does not represent a satisfactory solution to the problem.

Dry flushing may be stimulated by circulating vasoactive agents such as histamine and prostaglandins (produced endogenously). Antihistamine drugs, aspirin, and indomethicin are thus potential therapeutic agents for this type of flushing reaction. Alcohol and certain other drugs (such as nicotinic acid, amyl nitrite, opiates, and calcium channel blocking drugs) can also produce dry flushing. The application of tacrolimus and pimecrolimus to the face has been reported to induce intolerance to alcohol with sustained facial flushing (5). The flushing that occurs with the carcinoid syndrome, mastocytosis, and phaeochromocytoma is not usually accompanied by sweating and so fall into the category of "dry flushing."

Flushing accompanied by systemic symptoms (such as wheezing, palpitations, headache, diarrhea, weakness, weight loss) should alert the clinician to carry out appropriate investigations (see below) to determine if the patient has an underlying systemic disease such as carcinoid syndrome, mastocytosis, or phaeochromocytoma, all of which are rare causes of flushing.

The flush associated with the *carcinoid syndrome* has been classified into four different patterns. One pattern involves the face and chest and is relatively brief, lasting less than 5 minutes (Fig. 5).

Practice Point: This lady (Fig. 5) was referred for the management of frequent flushing that was thought to be related to rosacea. She appeared unwell, and a review of her medical history revealed that she suffered from episodes of diarrhoea and wheezing which were sometimes associated with the flushing. Flushing was extensive on the face and trunk. Investigations revealed the presence of elevated 5HIAA levels in the urine which confirmed the diagnosis of carcinoid syndrome.

Comment: Always take a comprehensive history on the first consultation with a patient complaining of frequent episodes of prolonged flushing. This will avoid many of the potential pitfalls of diagnosis and subsequent lack of response to therapy. If the case does not fit the diagnosis, go back over the patient's story. Asking the right question is the responsibility of the physician.

In other patients, the flush can be prolonged for more than 5 minutes. It is suggested that tumors originating in the embryonic foregut are more likely to provoke a "salmon pink" flush, while those originating in the midgut tend to produce a cyanotic hue. The flush in some patients can be quite dramatic, with an intense red flush extending diffusely over the face with involvement of the neck and upper chest which can last for hours or even days and be quite disabling. In others, the flush may produce a "geographic pattern" with bizarre gyrate or serpiginous patterns which tends to resolve centrally. In addition to the symptoms described above, the patients may experience edema and stiffness of the skin during flushing episodes and occasionally parasthesia of the fingers. Sclerodermoid features and skin changes caused by niacin deficiency (fragility, erythema, and hyperpigmentation) may also be seen in these patients. With successive attacks, the sclera may

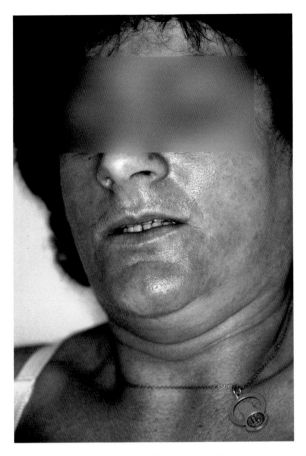

Figure 5 This patient has a flushing disorder secondary to the carcinoid syndrome. The picture shows extensive involvement on the face, neck, and upper chest. This patient also had extension of the flush area to the abdomen and back.

become injected in some patients and a permanent purplish or cyanotic hue develops in the distribution of the flush. This, in combination with the development of telangiectasias may give a plethoric appearance to the face that persists after the flush has cleared. The flush of the carcinoid syndrome may be precipitated in some patients by palpation of the abdomen or liver (if there are liver metastases), or by alcohol, emotional stress, sudden changes in temperature, or enemas.

Persistent edema and a "leonine facies" have been reported in a patient with longstanding carcinoid syndrome (6). This patient was reported to have "hypertrophic rosacea" and a biopsy of the skin revealed sebaceous hyperplasia with dermal scarring. These histological findings are similar to those seen in rhinophyma and the authors suggest that the frequent and prolonged episodes of flushing could be etiologically important in the genesis of this subtype of rosacea.

However, any association between the carcinoid syndrome and rosacea is open to question as reports of their concurrence appear to be no more common than would be expected by chance.

Degranulation of mast cells with flushing may occur in patients with *mastocytosis* after exercise, ingestion of alcohol, codeine, or injection of polymyxin B. Flushing in these patients may be accompanied by palpitations, diarrhea, and pruritus—the last of these symptoms being a useful clinical indicator. Dermatographia is often present in patients with mastocytosis which is a further helpful sign.

Hyperhidrosis, piloerection, and episodic hypertension in association with flushing can occur in patients with *phaeochromocytoma*. The flush often appears spontaneously and affects the face, neck, chest, and trunk. It lasts from 15 minutes to several hours and may be accompanied by sensations of profound weakness or even fainting attacks (7). A significant proportion of patients with phaeochromocytoma will in addition have the cutaneous stigmata of neurofibromatosis.

Flushing and severe pruritus or a burning sensation in the skin persisting for up to 30 minutes after a hot bath has been reported to be a feature of patients who have *polycythaemia* (either primary or secondary). Individuals with polycythemia vera often appear plethoric and have a ruddy complexion. This erythema, which may be associated with facial telangiectasias and fluctuate in intensity from time to time, can affect the face and neck but also the distal extremities, which helps to differentiate it from the facial erythema and telangiectasias seen in patients with rosacea. The veins of the sclera, retina, and oral mucosa may also be distended in patients with polycythemia.

Severe flushing has been reported to be the presenting feature of the *Zollinger-Ellison syndrome*. These patients may have a history of peptic ulcer disease and episodes of diarrhea caused by overproduction of the hormone gastrin by an islet cell tumor of the pancreas. *Bronchogenic carcinoma* and *medullary carcinoma of the thyroid* have also been reported to be associated with episodes of severe flushing in some patients.

Flushing after exercise can also occur with some forms of *cholinergic urticaria*. However, monosodium glutamate intolerance (*the "Chinese restaurant syndrome"*) appears not to be a true example of a flushing disorder. The propensity to flush vigorously after ingestion of alcohol is genetically determined by the deficiencies of the enzymes alcohol and aldehyde dehydrogenases. Alcohol-induced flushing appears to be more common amongst those of Chinese or Japanese (and North-American-Indian) origin, and is often provoked primarily by the alcohol. The flushing can reportedly be enhanced by chemical ingredients found in certain types or even brands of alcohol (gin, vodka, or lager are often blamed). Sodium nitrite, which is found in cured meats (frankfurters, bacon, salami, ham), may cause headache and flushing in some individuals.

Flushing, nausea and pain relieved by adopting an antiflexed position can occur in patients with horseshoe kidneys (*Rovsing syndrome*) (8) while unilateral

Table 1 Causes of Flushing

Emotion (blushing), anxiety, stress
Temperature (both hot and cold), sun exposure, fever, exercise, fluorescent lights
Foods, beverages, drugs, alcohol
Climacteric flushing
Rosacea
Neurologic (see below)
Carcinoid syndrome
Phaeochromocytoma
Mastocytosis
Polycythemia
Medullary carcinoma of thyroid
Renal carcinoma
Pancreatic cell tumor (VIP tumor)
Postsurgical (gastric/prostate/orchiectomy)
Anaphylaxis
Idiopathic

facial flushing with gustatory sweating may occur following parotid injury or surgery (*Frey's syndrome*).

DIFFERENTIAL DIAGNOSIS AND INVESTIGATIONS

See Algorithm 1 and Table 1.

An adequate medical history will reveal many of the causes of flushing such as the menopause in women and flushing in men after surgery for prostatic carcinoma who experience flushing and sweating symptoms similar to those in menopausal in women.

A detailed history will also reveal those patients who are food or alcohol sensitive and individuals who are taking drugs that are likely to precipitate flushing reactions (Table 2).

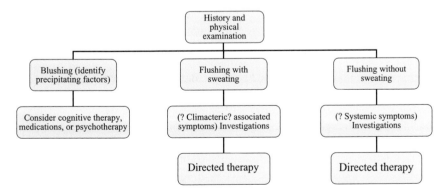

Algorithm 1   Algorithm for the initial evaluation of patients who present with flushing.

"Quod ali cibus est aliis fuat acre venenum"—
What is food to one is bitter poison to others"
Lucretius (99–55 B.C.)

A recent described example of a topical agent capable of inducing flushing is 0.1% tacrolimus ointment. Intolerance to alcohol with sustained facial flushing occurs in up to 7% of adult patients exposed to this agent. Flushing is not confined to the treated areas, but is limited by anatomic boundaries such as the hairline, the tip of the nose and the base of the neck. The mechanism of this reaction is unknown, but release of neuropeptides such as substance P with vasodilatory properties has been suggested. Niacin, a drug that is usually prescribed for its lipid lowering properties, causes prolonged flushing in up to 80% of patients. It appears to activate Langerhan cells to produce and release prostaglandin (PGD2) which binds to a specific receptor on dermal blood vessels and causes vascular muscle relaxation and vasodilatation.

A history of gastric surgery may explain why a patient has developed flushing, tachycardia, sweating, weakness, and gastrointestinal upset (the "dumping syndrome"). This reaction is often provoked by a meal or ingestion of hot fluids or hypertonic glucose.

The precipitating or provoking agents of flushing should be listed for each patient and they should be asked to keep a diary of events to identify potential triggers. This will help to classify the type of flushing that they suffer from and guide management.

These patient records sometimes can give useful information as to causation (e.g., flushing after food, alcohol, a hot bath, or exercise as outlined above), and are also important in the management. Identifying these "triggers" enables the physician to develop a strategy of avoidance for the future (Tables 3 and 4).

A history of *neurologic problems* [(migraine, brain tumors, and Parkinson disease, etc. (Table 5)] may explain the basis of flushing reactions in some patients.

As mentioned above, patients who have systemic symptoms such as wheezing or dyspnoea, headache, palpitations, weakness,or episodes of profound anxiety associated with flushing, diarrhea, or weight loss should have additional investigations carried out. These may be carried out in consultation with appropriate specialists and include monitoring of blood pressure (for both carcinoid syndrome and phaeochromocytoma), a full blood count and serum iron levels (sometimes polycythemia rubra vera or polycythema secondary to hemochromocytosis can give rise to facial erythema or flushing), skin biopsy for mastocytosis (although the histologic changes may be subtle and increased mast cell numbers difficult to demonstrate even with the use of special stains), abdominal ultrasound (for both the carcinoid syndrome and phaeochromocytoma as well as to rule out horseshoe kidneys and other organ abnormalities), and additional scanning investigations as appropriate in the clinical setting, 24 hour urine collection for 5 hydroxyindole acetic acid (HIAA) or measurement of circulating levels of serotonin (carcinoid syndrome) vanillylmandelic acid (VMA) (phaeochromocytoma) and histamine products for mastocytosis (Table 6). A bone marrow biopsy may also be required

Table 2 Drugs That May Induce Flushing: (Partial List)

A. Spontaneously
 Vasodilators (e.g., nitroglycerin)
 Calcium channel blockers (e.g., nifedipine)
 Angiotensin converting enzyme inhibitors
 Oral or intrasynovial triamcinolone
 High-dose pulse methylprednisolone
 Nicotinic acid (block flush with asprin/indomethicin)
 Morphine and other opiates
 Amyl and butyl nitrite (recreational drugs)
 Metrifonate (block flush with atropine)
 Bromocriptine /Cholinergic drugs
 Tamoxifen
 Vancomycin
 Rifampin
 Thyrotropin-releasing hormone
 Calcitonin gene-related peptide
 Cyproterone acetate (also used for postorchiectomy patients)
 Cyclosporin A (tacrolimus may provide an alternative)
 Prostaglandins D2, E, NSAIDs
 Combination anaesthesia with isoflurane and fentanyl
 Contrast media
 Caffeine withdrawl

B. With alcohol
 Antimalarials
 Disulfiram
 Chlorpropamide
 Calcium carbamide
 Phentolamine
 Griseofulvin
 Metronidazole
 Ketoconazole
 Tacrolimus ointment (7% of patients report flushing reactions)
 Cefamandole
 Cefoperazone
 Moxalactam
 Benorylate
 Trichloroethylene (solvent) in occupational degreasers
 N,N-Dimethylferamide
 N-Butylaldoxiam}
 Xylene or carbon disulfide occupational exposure

Table 3   Foods and Drinks Likely to Cause Flushing

Hot foods (especially in large quantities)
Spicy foods (especially chili peppers and histamine rich foods)
Hot drinks (tea, coffee, hot water)
Won ton soup (monosodium glutamate)
Coffee or caffeine containing drinks (or caffeine withdrawl)
Alcohol (especially if alcohol dehydrogenase deficient)
Fruits (especially lemons)
Vegetables (mushrooms and histamine rich)
Meats (Sodium nitrite in frankfurters, bacon and ham and histamine rich)
Fish (histamine/cigua toxin)
Dairy products (cheese and chocolate and histamine rich)

Table 4   Histamine-Rich Foods and Drinks

Cheeses (Parmesan, blue, Roquefort, Monterey Jack)
Vegetables (eggplant, spinach, tomato)
Meats (salami, chicken, chicken liver)
Wines (Chianti, Burgundy)

Table 5   Neurologic Flushing

Anxiety
Emotion (Blushing)
Brain tumors
Spinal cord lesions
Orthostatic hypotension
Migraine headaches
Parkinson disease

Table 6   Investigations

Careful History (drugs, foods, other illness, associated symptoms, etc.)
Blood count, renal, liver profiles
Urinalysis
Abdominal CT scan (if considering systemic cause)
Carcinoid—24 hr urine for 5 HIAA, whole blood serotonin
Phaeochromocytoma—plasma or urine catecholamine and metanephrines
Mastocytosis—24 hr urine histamine, bone marrow examination

to establish the diagnosis of mastocytosis. Skin biopsies are not usually helpful in distinguishing the different types of flush or blush reaction.

KEY POINTS

- A tendency to frequent flushing in teenagers rarely implies an underlying disorder.
- The prognosis in this age group is usually good as flushing frequency typically decreases with age.
- Flushing accompanied by sweating implies autonomic nervous system involvement.
- Flushing in a patient with symptoms of wheezing, palpitations, diarrhoea etc indicates a need for systemic work-up.
- A diary of dietary and alcohol intake and factors related to episodes of flushing can be useful for both the patient and the clinician.

MANAGEMENT

The management of the patient who presents with troublesome recurrent and prolonged episodes of flushing or blushing begins with a *detailed history* to identify the type of reaction taking place, the associated features (sweating, etc.), and any *precipitating or exacerbating factors* or situations as well as any actions or agents that relieve the problem. Particular attention should be paid to the *drug history* as there are several medications and other agents which may cause flushing (Table 2). The avoidance of these and other identified precipitating agents such as foods and beverages (Table 3), particularly those containing histamine (Table 4) is an obvious necessity as is the requirement to ensure that the work *environment is not overheated*, the *humidity* is finely adjusted, and *strong sunlight is avoided*.

The diagnosis of blushing is made on the history and individuals with disorders of blushing are often sensitive, shy and introverted by nature. Such individuals may benefit from *psychotherapy and cognitive behavior therapy* to desensitize them to the triggering social situations. Some of these patients may also benefit from *low dosage beta-blockers* which have the effect of reducing the reactive tachycardia and tremor which is sometimes present and are mildly anxiolytic as well. Fatigue and dizziness are potential side effects of beta-blocker therapy. If the anxiety overlay is significant then consideration should be given to the use of other *anxiolytic agents* in the short term. Female patients often appreciate expert advice on cosmetic cover to maximize the camouflage of their embarrassing redness (see chap. 8). Other drugs (Table 7) have been used to treat flushing patients with reports of successful outcomes in individual patients or small groups. It must be recognized that the use of these drugs for flushing is off-label so the patient should be appropriately advised and caution exercised in their use. Initiation of therapy at low dosages in most instances is recommended and as tolerance is

Table 7 Management of Flushing

Identify and treat cause when possible
Identify and avoid precipitating/provoking factors
Consider counseling or cognitive behavior therapy
Cosmetic cover and cooling techniques
Topical oxymetazoline
Drugs
   Aspirin (blocks nicotinic acid flush)
   Antihistamines (H_1 and H_2)
   Anxiolytics (for anxiety related blushing)
   Beta-blockers (propranolol, nadolol)
   Alpha blockers (clonidine hydrochloride)
   Indomethacin
HRT/progestagens/venlafaxine/paroxetine/fluoxetine/gabapentin
   Diclofenac sodium (postmenopause)
   Diethylstilbestrol (postorchiectomy)
   Cyproterone acetate (postorchiectomy)
   Naloxone (flushing with organic psychosis)
   Pyridoxine (for glutamate mediated flushing)
   Botulinum toxin injection
Surgery (endoscopic transthoracic sympathectomy)
Laser therapy
Herbal therapies
Homeopathy
Other (hypnotherapy, acupuncture, naturotherapy)

---

demonstrated the dosage can be increased. Topical *oxymetazoline* has recently been reported to be successful in treating the erythema and flushing in a small number of patients with rosacea (9). *Botulinum toxin A intradermal injection* for neck and facial blushing has been reported in isolated patients, but the beneficial effect (if any) is likely to be short lived and further studies are needed before this form of treatment can be recommended. *Bilateral endoscopic transthoracic sympathectomy* has been reported to be helpful in the majority of a large group of patients with uncontrollable facial blushing which was having serious detrimental effects on their social, occupational, or sexual lives (10). However, there can be serious side effects to such intervention including pneumothorax, haemorrhage, and postsurgical compensatory hyperhidrosis in a significant number of patients.

Postmenopausal flushing is often markedly diminished with the introduction of *HRT*. For those unable to take this medication or unwilling to do so, *clonidine, venlafaxine, and gabapentin* have been reported to be helpful in the management of this type of flush reaction. Herbal treatments are often used to treat post-menopausal flushing. *Red clover and soy isoflavones* or plant phytoestrogens were thought to be helpful, but objective evidence is lacking. Vitamin E has also been suggested as an effective treatment, but studies have failed to show a significantly beneficial effect. Black cohosh, ginseng, liquorice root, sage, and sarsaparilla are unconventional remedies that have been recommended for menopausal flushing without firm scientific basis. *Acupuncture* has been reported as being helpful in one study, possibly by increasing the hypothalamic beta-endorphin activity. Hypnotherapy and naturopathic remidies have been recommended for patients with flushing and in the absence of effective medical therapy have been used by many people. Unfortunately the results of such treatments have not been scientifically evaluated.

Male postorchiectomy patients may benefit from treatment with *diethylstilbestrol* or the anti androgen *cyproterone acetate*.

REFERENCES

1. Wilkin JK. Epigastric rosacea. Arch Derm. 1980; 116:584.
2. Darwin C. The Expression of the emotions in man and animals. London, UK: John Murray, 1872.
3. Stearns V, Ullmer L, Lopez JF, et al. Hot flushes. Lancet 2002; 360:1851–1861.
4. Sterns V Clinical update: New treatments for hot flushes. Lancet 2007; 369:2062–2064.
5. Milingou M, Antille C, Sorg O, et al. Alcohol intolerance and facial flushing in patients treated with topical tacrolimus. Arch Derm 2004; 140:1542–1544.
6. Findlay GH, Simson IW. Leonine hypertrophic rosacea associated with a benign bronchial. Tumor Clin Expt Dermatol 1977; 2:175–176.
7. Lenders JW, Eisenhofer G, Mannelli M, et al. Phaeochromocytoma. Lancet 2005; 366:665–672.
8. Mooney E. The flushing patient. Int J Dermatol 1985; 24:549–554.
9. Shanler SD, Ondo AL. Successful treatment of the erythema and flushing of rosacea using a topically applied selective alpha-1 adrenergic receptor agonist, oxymetazoline. Arch Dermatol 2007; 143:1369–1371.
10. Drott C, Cales G, Ollson-Rex L, et al. Successful treatment of facial blushing by endoscopic transthoracic sympathectomy. Brit J Dermatol 1998; 138:639–643.

FURTHER READING

Burgess TH. The Physiology or Mechanism of Blushing. London, UK: John Churchill, 1839.
Comment: If you can get your hands on a reprint or copy of this book, you will be able to absorb yourself in an excellent thesis on this subject replete with references to plants and other living organisms!

Shelly WB, Shelly ED. Advanced Dermatologic Therapy II. WB Saunders Company 2001.
Comment: This is a wonderful book, the one to go to when searching for inspiration in the management of the difficult case. Beautifully written with inspiring anecdotes by this team of great dermatologists, the chapter on flushing is particularly well worth consulting.

3

The Classification and Grading of Severity of Rosacea

"...rosacea, a nice name for an unpleasant complaint..."
John Banville (The Sea)

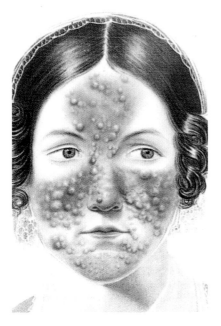

Figure 1   This beautifully executed drawing from the 1800's clearly illustrates the clinical features of papulopustular rosacea (PPR). Note the central distribution of inflammatory lesions on the face, the contrasting pallor of the normal skin (particularly around the eyes) and the papulopustular morphology of the eruption. The artist has even captured the anxious distressed look on this unfortunate woman's face confronted with this disfiguring facial rash.

To understand the basis for the classification of rosacea into subtypes, it is necessary to first look back at the historical development of the concept of rosacea as a disease entity. Over time, the term "rosacea" was applied to several different clinical entities that had in common redness of the face. It is illuminating to review how early practitioners viewed this disorder and important to realize that until an etiology or etiologies are shown to cause one or other of the various subtypes of rosacea concepts regarding what constitutes this disorder will continue to evolve.

HISTORICAL BACKGROUND

Rosacea was originally described in exacting detail by one of the most prominent doctors of his time, the English dermatologist Robert Willan (1757–1812). He practiced at the Carey Street dispensary in London, one of the first institutions to focus on diseases of the skin. Willan's description of rosacea was published one year after his death by his pupil and former colleague Bateman in a seminal publication on the classification of diseases of the skin in 1813. The term "acne rosacea" was introduced into the medical literature and the disease was defined as a dermatosis which was distinctive from acne vulgaris occurring in an older age group but which shared some similarities with that disorder. Willan chose the term "acne rosacea" to convey both the similarity to acne vulgaris (the presence of multiple erythematous facial papules and pustules), but also to highlight another characteristic of the disorder, i.e., the striking reddened appearance of the facial skin which distinguished it from acne vulgaris (Figure 1). This differentiation was further delineated by Willan's fellow countryman Erasmus Wilson (1809–1884) in 1842 when he suggested the possibility of a common pathogenic pathway for acne rosacea and acne vulgaris. In those early days, acne rosacea was considered to be a skin condition closely related to acne vulgaris in both its clinical presentation and pathogenesis. In support of this thinking, the great French dermatologist Jean-Louis Alibert (1768–1837) cited a postmortem study by his colleague in Alphonse Devergie (1798–1879) in Hopital Saint Louis, Paris, France. The latter studied the pathologic changes in a patient with "gutta rosacea" and reported that the pathogenic process in rosacea involved the sebaceous glands. Alibert studied many patients with this disorder (Figure 2) and classified rosacea in the group of dermatoses with sebaceous gland pathologies (which included acne vulgaris), and observed the concurrence of comedones (blocked openings of the sebaceous glands) in some patients. This hypothesis of sebaceous gland dysfunction in rosacea was also supported by Paul Gerson Unna (1850–1929), a German physician who practiced in Hamburg and who was regarded as one of the foremost dermatologists of early decades of the 20th century.

However, some English dermatologists of the early 20th century, particularly Radcliff-Crocker (1845–1909), considered the term "acne rosacea" to be inappropriate. They argued that the redness of acne rosacea was not due to inflammation of the pilosebaceous glands or blockage of their follicles, but instead postulated that it was due to an abnormal dilatation of the blood vessels of the face. They

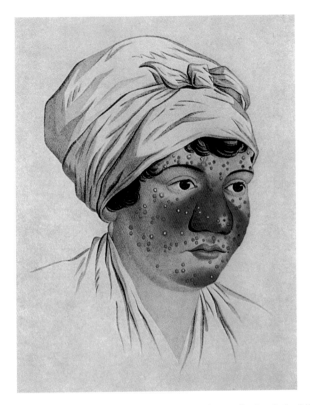

Figure 2 Another wonderful example of a medical artist's skill in representing and deliberately exaggerating the detailed clinical features of PPR in this portrait of a French patient from the nineteenth century. The different hairstyles and attire convey a definite sense of the personality of the individual illustrated. Note the prominence of the nose suggesting early rhinophyma, an uncommon occurrence in a female patient.

recommended that the prefix "acne" be dropped and that the condition be simply known as "rosacea," a disorder different in every way from acne vulgaris. In this regard, they were probably recognizing the subtype we now know as erythematotelangiectatic rosacea (ETTR - see chapter 4) as well as the fact that many patients with rosacea complain of heat intolerance and have a tendency to flush. Radcliff-Crocker and his colleagues proposed that rosacea was due to hyperreactivity of the facial vessels manifested by frequent flushing. They suggested that the repeated dilatation of the facial blood vessels, initially followed by constriction, ultimately lead to a situation where these vessels remained permanently dilated with consequent chronic congestion (telangiectasias). They postulated that these widened and lax vessel walls with sluggish congested blood flow leaked fluid into the perivascular dermal tissue. The leaked material caused a reactive inflammation in the skin surrounding the vessels giving rise to the lesions of papulopustular

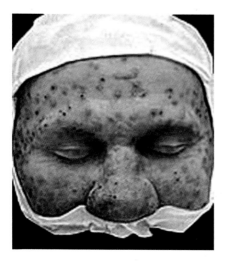

Figure 3 Wax models (moulages) of patient's skin diseases were used before photography was readily available and allowed students to study skin disorders in color and in a three dimensional fashion. This moulage shows a middle-aged male patient with widespread PPR and early rhinophyma.

rosacea (PPR see chapter 5). They also proposed that the chronic congestion of the facial vessels ultimately lead to the hypertrophic tissue changes of phymatous rosacea (PR - see chapter 6), which was regarded as "end-stage rosacea." This theory thus proposed that rosacea progressed in stages from frequent flushing to fixed dilated blood vessels (erythematotelangiectatic rosacea), followed by the development of papules and pustules (PPR) and ultimately in the final expression of the disorder, the endpoint of phymatous change PR. However, convenient as this theory was in providing an encompassing pathogenesis for every expression of rosacea it ignored the reality that not all patients with rosacea complained of frequent flushing. In patients who complained of flushing this was not always the first symptom preceding all other changes as they suggested. In addition, telangiectasias were not always a feature of the clinical picture of PPR and some patients with prominent telangiectasias never developed papules or pustules. Finally, some individuals who developed phymatous changes (especially rhinophyma) had mild or even no previous history of inflammatory rosacea or preceding flushing.

Rosacea-like Eruption

Over the years, several other clinical entities were incorporated under the broadening rubric of rosacea. These included "**granulomatous rosacea,**" also known as "lupus miliaris disseminatus faciei" or "Lewandowski's disease". This is a chronic eruption of reddish dome shaped papules on the face which were composed of granulomas when examined histologically and which were resistant to most forms of therapy. The relationship (if any) of this eruption to other manifestations of rosacea is unclear, and in the classification of rosacea, it was suggested that patients with these eruptions be regarded as having a variant of the disease rather than a subtype.

Another condition suggested to be a form of rosacea was "**rosacea conglobata,**" a dramatic eruption of large cystic lesions accompanied by marked facial erythema which occurred mostly in young women. This disorder could have a devastating cosmetic effect in the inflammatory stages and was often followed by scarring. Rosacea Conglobata had been formerly described under the title of "**pyoderma faciale**" and had been considered as a form of acne vulgaris, but the intense erythema which accompanied the eruption suggested to some dermatologists that it should be reclassified as a form of rosacea. However, because of its deep cystic and scarring nature (unlike other forms of rosacea), it was thought premature to include it as a subtype or variant of rosacea without further evidence of its pathogenesis. For a clear description of this dermatosis, the reader is referred to the excellent textbook by Plewig and Kligman mentioned earlier.

Other diseases which were included in the rosacea spectrum under such terms as "**rosacea fulminans**" (an explosive onset of a generalized pustular eruption of the face with erythema), and "**prerosacea**" for some of those individuals who suffered from frequent flushing and sensitive skin but without any other stigmata of rosacea. Because this diagnosis could only be made with certainty after the development of inflammatory changes this term was not recommended by the classification group. "**Steroid-induced rosacea**" and "rosacea-like dermatosis" were other terms used for the eruption of facial erythema, papules, and pustules induced by various medications. "**Demodecosis**" and "**pityriasis folliculorum**" were thought to be conditions closely related to rosacea and characterized by tiny superficial papules, pustules, and prominent surface scaling with associated erythema. These eruptions are accompanied by a marked proliferation in the numbers of demodex folliculorum mites on the face which can be demonstrated by gently scraping the skin surface with a glass slide and examining the scale under a microscope a medium power (see chapter 5).

It is clear from the above review that the concept of the disease described by Willan had changed markedly as time progressed. Because such a wide diversity of dermatoses was included under the term "rosacea" clinicians became increasingly confused as to which entity within the rosacea spectrum was being described in investigative studies. The epidemiologic studies as well as retrospective reviews of the clinical and histologic features of large numbers of patients carried out in different academic centers had results that were often conflicting and difficult to interpret, and their relevance to the understanding of the pathogenesis of rosacea uncertain.

The lack of precise definition of the various subtypes of rosacea and the poorly based assumption that rosacea was a disorder that progressed from flushing to phymatous changes required that a new classification of the clinical components which constituted the essential features of the disease be undertaken without including any preconceived notion of its pathogenic progression or stages of evolution.

THE CLASSIFICATION OF ROSACEA

In 2002 a group of dermatologists under the auspices of the National Rosacea Society (U.S.) came together to develop a classification of rosacea that would allow for the easy identification of the various clinical subtypes of the disorder without implying a pathogenesis or progression of the disorder through various stages (1). Following prolonged discussion, it became clear that there were four clinical subtypes of the disorder that could be readily identified by their clinical characteristics.

Subtype 1, Erythematotelangiectatic rosacea (ETTR), was characterized by persistent central facial erythema, frequent flushing, and often the presence of multiple facial telangiectasias. ETTR was recognized to be an entity in its own right, but it could also serve as the background on which subtype 2, papulopustular rosacea (PPR) arose. Patients with ETTR had sensitive facial skin which was reactive to temperature change and the overlap with heliodermatitis was recognized. PPR was recognized by the presence of multiple small bright erythematous dome-shaped papules and papulopustules which appeared in crops on the central facial skin (nose, central forehead, and chin as well as medial cheeks). Some of the individuals with PPR also complained of a tendency to flush frequently and some had the background changes of ETTR as described. Subtype 3 was called phymatous rosacea (PR) and encompassed those patients who developed persistent nonpainful non pitting facial swelling associated with erythema. In some of these patients, the swelling was preceded by or accompanied other manifestations of rosacea (such as ETTR or PPR) but in others the persistent swelling arose de novo. The most easily recognized type of PR is rhinophyma where the nose becomes progressively enlarged and distorted as a result of overgrowth of sebaceous glands and connective tissue. Swelling of areas such as the forehead (mentophyma), chin (gnathophyma), ears (otophyma), and eyelids (blepharophyma) were identified separately and may have a different genesis as their histopathology is not the same as that seen in rhinophyma. The fourth subtype identified (subtype 4) was ocular rosacea (OR). This recognized the common finding of ocular changes in patients with rosacea. These changes were usually mild and nonspecific (such as dryness of the eyes, blepharitis, or conjunctivitis) and were difficult to diagnose as being related to rosacea in the absence of the characteristic skin lesions. Meibomian gland dysfunction seemed to be a particularly common finding in rosacea patients (Table 1). In forming this classification it was recognized by the expert group that there was potential for clinical overlap between subtypes, and that individual patients could manifest more than one subtype simultaneously (for example, ETTR and PPR, or PPR and OR). Although the subtypes were numbered from one to four, this was not intended to imply a progression of the disorder form one subtype to another, and it was

Table 1   The Subtypes of Rosacea (3)

Subtype (number/name)	Clinical characteristics
Subtype 1: ETTR	Persistent central facial erythema, frequent flushing, may be telangiectatic vessels
Subtype 2: PPR	Erythematous dome-shaped papules, some with surmounting pustulation in a centrofacial distribution on a background of persistent erythema
Subtype 3: PR	Persistent facial swelling with hypertrophy of tissue (rhinophyma); different variants described
Subtype 4: OR	Ocular inflammation (blepharritis/conjunctivitis/meibomian gland dysfunction/chalazion, etc.)

accepted that each subtype might potentially have a separate pathogenic mechanism and that they might even represent separate entities within in the rosacea spectrum.

Although this classification had limitations (2), it represented an important step toward the rationalization of what had become a mélange of clinical entities. For the first time since Willan's original description of the disorder, clinicians were able to use a widely accepted definition of what constituted this disorder and communication between investigators was facilitated by common recognition of which subtype within the rosacea spectrum that they were studying. The classification also facilitated management of patients by clinicians as the therapeutic choices were largely dictated by which subtype of rosacea the patient had.

THE GRADING OF SEVERITY OF ROSACEA

The grading of rosacea was undertaken to formulate a common system of ranking of the degree of severity of each subtype in order to facilitate comparison of investigative studies from different academic centers as well as to provide the clinician treating a patient with rosacea with a practical tool to evaluate their response to therapeutic intervention (4).

The terms used in the grading of rosacea were necessarily broad (mild, moderate, and severe) but served as guidelines for the purposes outlined above (Table 2). With improved methods of measuring parameters in the skin such as erythema, lesion size and number, area of involvement, skin swelling, and ocular gland function, this grading system will be superseded by more accurate evaluation of disease severity of each subtype.

In the following chapters, we will discuss each of the rosacea subtypes in turn looking at their definition, distribution, clinical features, histopathology, differential diagnosis, and management options.

Table 2   Grading of Severity of Subtypes of Rosacea (4)

Subtype	Mild	Moderate	Severe
Subtype 1: ETTR	Mild persistent facial erythema	Moderate persistent erythema	Severe erythema
	Mild tendency to flush	Frequent flushing	Frequent prolonged flushing
	May be scattered telangiectasias	Telangiectasias present	Many telangiectias
Subtype 2: PPR	Few papules/ pustules	Several papules/ pustules	Many papules/ pustules-may be plaques studded with lesions
	Mild erythema	Moderate erythema	Pronounced erythema
Subtype 3: PR (grading applies to rhinophyma)	Dilated nasal pores (patulous follicles) with mild nasal swelling	Bulbous nasal swelling/mild tissue/hypertrophy	Marked nasal swelling
			Tissue hypertrophy with nasal distortion
Subtype 4: OR	Mild dryness/itch	Burning/stinging	Pain/photosensitivity
	Mild conjunctival injection	Blepharritis/chalazion or hordeolum	Severe lid changes/ corneal changes/ episcleritis
		Moderate conjunctival injection	

KEY POINTS

- The original descriptions of "acne rosacea" referred to what is now known as papulopustular rosacea (Subtype 2).
- Early dermatologists felt rosacea was a disorder related to sebaceous gland dysfunction.
- The inclusion of several different disorders under the term rosacea included a large spectrum of clinical entities.
- The classification of rosacea into subtypes is intended to facilitate the understanding of the disease and guide clinicians to appropriate therapies.
- Grading of severity of rosacea is also helpful in choosing appropriate treatments and in evaluation of the response to therapy.

REFERENCES

1. Wilkin J, Dahl M, Detmar M, et al. Standard classification of rosacea: Report of the National Rosacea Society Expert Committee on the Classification and Staging of Rosacea. J Am Acad Dermatol 2002; 46:584–587.
2. Crawford GH, Pelle MT, James WD. Rosacea: Etiology, pathogenesis and subtype classification. J Am Acad Dermatol 2004; 51:327–341.
3. Berg M, Linden S. An epidemiological study of rosacea. Acta Derm Venereol 1989; 69:419–423.
4. Wilkin J, Dahl M, Detmar M, et al. Standard grading system for rosacea: Report of the National Rosacea Society Expert Committee on the Classification and Staging of Rosacea. J Am Acad Dermatol 2004; 50:907–912.

4

Subtype 1 Erythematotelangiectatic Rosacea

"I never think of your face but I think upon hell fire. . . ."
Shakespeare, *(Henry IV)*

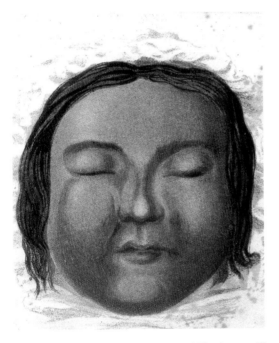

Figure 1   This illustration from the 1800s shows a 30-year-old patient with erythema and congestive swelling of the face secondary to her third attack of "erysipelas idiopathicum" which was thought at the time to be caused by "exposure to cold." Erysipelas is now known to be a bacterial infection of the skin which may cause severe debility with facial redness and swelling. Erysipelas may occasionally be mistaken for erythematotelangiectatic rosacea.

DEFINITION

Erythematotelangiectatic rosacea (ETTR) is characterized by persistent facial erythema with a tendency to repeated and prolonged episodes of facial flushing often with the appearance of multiple telangiectatic vessels in the affected facial skin (1).

DISTRIBUTION

Patients with established subtype 1 rosacea have facial erythema that extends from the dorsum of the nose across the central face to involve the medial and central cheeks, stopping just short of the auricular tragus. It is usually limited from below by the inferior margin of the mandibular ramus and from above by the superior aspect of the malar bones (Figs. 2 and 3). The central areas of the forehead and chin may also be affected.

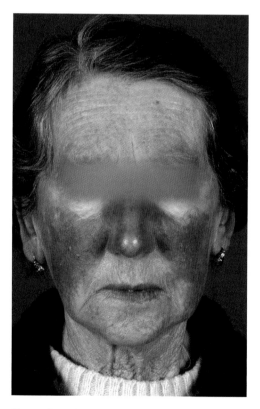

Figure 2   This woman has the typical facial distribution of erythema and telangiectasias of ETTR. Note involvement of the bridge of the nose and the profound persistent erythema extending across the medial cheeks and sparing under the eyes and nose. The forehead is spared in this patient, an area often affected by those individuals who have erythema and telangiectasias as a result of chronic actinic damage (heliodermatitis).

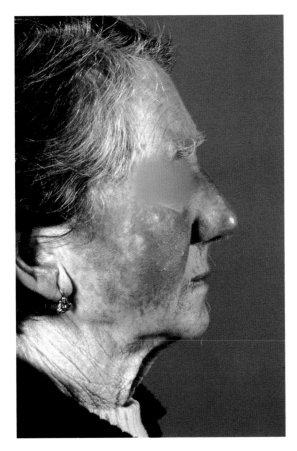

Figure 3 The involvement of the lateral cheeks with profound persistent erythema and telangiectasias is shown in this patient with ETTR. The neck is not involved again helping in the distinction from heliodermatitis.

BACKGROUND

The concept of ETTR as a subtype of rosacea grew out of the recognition of the essential constituents of the clinical picture of rosacea, i.e., the persistent facial redness, a tendency to frequent flushing in some patient and the frequent presence of multiple fixed dilated small blood vessels (telangiectasias) on the face. The term ETTR has been used to describe the clinical picture produced by the combination of these skin changes. Photodamage is recognized to be an important element both in the production and exacerbation of ETTR (from clinical and histologic evidence), but whether it is the determining factor in its pathogenesis is unclear at this time (2).

It has been argued that cutaneous features similar to ETTR are the main clinical findings in patients with heliodermatitis. Heliodermatitis is a descriptive term recently introduced to describe the clinical features produced by repeated

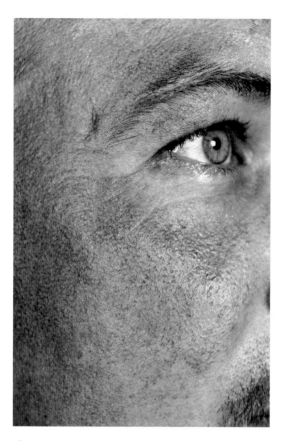

Figure 4   This outdoor worker (farmer) shows the typical skin changes caused by actinic damage sustained by a sun-sensitive individual. This becomes evident after repeated climatic exposure over many years (heliodermatitis). The erythema and telangiectasias are distributed generally over the facial skin with accentuation on the prominences.

sun exposure on the facial skin of sun-sensitive individuals (3). Individuals with fair skin types 1 or 2, often with blue or gray eyes, red or blond hair, sunburn easily as outlined in chapter 1. In time and with repeated ultraviolet light wind and cold exposure (often occupational or recreational), these people may develop facial erythema that persists after the initiating stimulus has passed as well as multiple small- to medium-sized fixed dilated blood vessels in the most exposed areas, i.e., the facial convexities (forehead, cheeks, nose, and chin). Such changes have been recognized by the general public for many years, and the terms "Farmers Face" or "Fisherman's Face" have been used to describe them in recognition of the climatic influence in producing these features (Fig. 4). Sometimes a redness of the neck is also seen in these individuals giving rise to the term "red neck" as used to be applied to rural outdoor workers. The overlap of clinical features of ETTR and heliodermatitis make the differentiation between these conditions problematic, and as a result some clinicians use the terms interchangeably.

> **Practice Point**: The farmer in Figure 4 had skin type 1 and was referred because his "rosacea" would not respond to topical metronidazole gel (it caused stinging) or doxycycline orally for six weeks (it made no impact on the redness). His history of prolonged climatic exposure, the widespread distribution of erythema and telangiectasias (including to his neck) and his type 1 skin suggested that a diagnosis of heliodermatitis was likely. He was advised on sun protection (Daily all year round application of a high factor sun block cream and wearing a hat), and his telangiectasias were treated with intense pulsed-light laser.
> *Comment: It is often difficult to distinguish clinically between subtype 1 rosacea and heliodermatitis. However, the management of both conditions is similar. These patients have skin that is poorly tolerant of topical medications and systemic therapy has no effect on the redness.*

Individuals who have ETTR or heliodermatitis are equally sensitive to fluctuations in ambient temperature. In particular, a warm environment can trigger a rapid increase in their facial erythema in the form of a flush, which may be sustained for prolonged periods. A similar flushing effect may be produced by the ingestion of hot drinks, spicy foods, or a large hot meal. Alcohol (red wine and beer are often cited as being the main culprits by sufferers) can also produce this effect.

In addition, persons with ETTR or heliodermatitis have sensitive, easily irritated skin that is abnormally reactive to minor skin stimulants. Perfumated facial products such as after-shave lotions, air fresheners, or sprays (such as antiperspirants) tend to cause a burning or stinging sensation in the affected skin. Minor variations in humidity and level of air conditioning may also cause facial irritation in such patients (Table 1) (4). Exposure of the facial skin to strong or cold wind often leads to a sensation of intense discomfort almost amounting to pain. The bright erythema may take on a dusky blue purple or violaceous hue as the individual gets older and the telangiectatic vessels dilate giving a "cyanotic" appearance (Fig. 5). Occasionally patients will have splayed telangiectatic vessels at the sides and on the bridge of the nose without marked erythema. The precise classification of these eruptions is unclear, but in time they often develop increasing erythema, and some patients (especially males) seem to be prone to changes of rhinophyma (Figures 6, 7). In others the telangiectatic components is prominently visible on the cheeks with a varying degree of accompanying erythema (Figure 8). The color of the nose may vary according to the ambient temperature, appearing red in warm weather and bluish in colder weather.

> *". . . his nose . . . is like a coal of fire, . . . sometimes blue and sometimes red."*
> Shakespeare, *(King Henry V)*

Even though ETTR is classified as subtype 1 rosacea, this is not intended to suggest that it represents the first stage in the progressive development of the

Table 1 Factors Flaring ETTR

Alcohol (especially red wine and beer)
Hot beverages (heat is critical but not presence of caffeine)
Hot meals (especially in large volumes or with spices)
Exposure to sunlight (applies all year around)
Exposure to wind (especially harsh cold winds)
Perfumed facial products and those containing sorbic acid
Astringents and cleansers containing acetone or alcohol
Abrasive or exfoliant facial preparations
Facial massage or vigorous rubbing
Toners or moisturisers containing glycolic acid
Drugs that cause or exacerbate flushing (see chap. 2)
Hot, humid environments (saunas, hot tubs, etc.)
Strenuous exercise (particularly in a warm climate)
Psychologic stress and emotional upset

Patients should keep a diary to identify factors that cause exacerbation of their skin condition as there is considerable individual variation of the factors that flare ETTR.

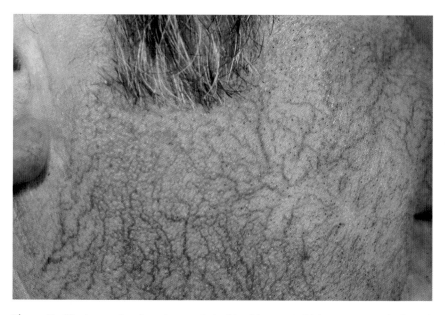

Figure 5 The large telangiectatic vessels in this older man which course over the lateral cheeks have developed a bluish cyanotic hue that becomes more marked on exposure to cold. Large vessels such as these are often attributed to chronic ultraviolet light exposure. Note impressive background erythema that was persistent suggesting the diagnosis of ETTR.

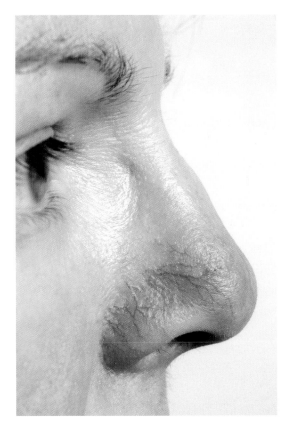

Figure 6 Small telangiectatic vessels are visible on the side of the nose in this young woman with ETTR. Localized aggregation of vessels such as these may occur as an isolated finding without features of ETTR elsewhere on the face. Such vessels usually respond readily to laser therapy.

other subtypes of rosacea and many patients do not subsequently develop other manifestations of rosacea. The inflammatory papules and pustules of stage 2 (papulopustular) rosacea (PPR) do not develop as a consequence of the erythema and telangiectasias in subtype 1 disease. In fact, while the cutaneous changes of PPR may indeed develop on a background of photodamage (as would be expected in a cohort of middle aged sun sensitive individuals) the telangiectasias characteristically seen in subtype 2 rosacea are often finer than those seen in individuals with ETTR or heliodermatitis. Typically the erythema associated with PPR is secondary to inflammatory changes in the skin rather than the presence of telangiectatic vessels (Fig. 9).

Thus, while some doubt surrounds the nosology of the skin changes in patients classified as having either ETTR or heliodermatitis, and while the relationship of these changes to the other subtypes of rosacea is disputed, it is useful

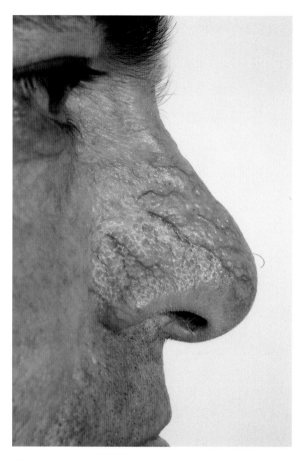

Figure 7   This young man has more prominent telangiectatic vessels which course across the sides of the nose giving it a marked erythematous color, especially in a warm environment. The adverse cosmetic impact was considerable. Note the prominent "patulous" follicles suggesting the early development of rhinophyma.

from the clinicians' perspective to group these patients together. They share common clinical features, have similar factors that irritate their sensitive skin, and require the same types of therapeutic interventions. The term ETTR will be used henceforth to describe these individuals.

CLINICAL FEATURES

Patients with ETTR have a striking clinical appearance. In its fully developed form there is profound erythema of the central face with accentuation on the projecting skin surfaces. The depth of erythema ranges from faint pink/red at the periphery of the cheeks to a deep burgundy color of the central face

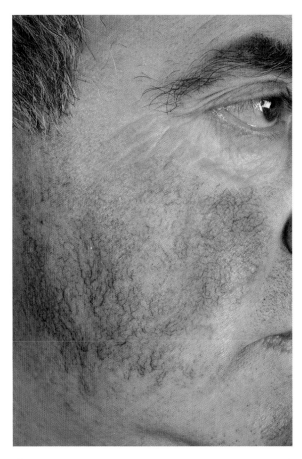

Figure 8 Involvement of the medial and lateral cheeks with marked telangiectasias and a degree of erythema is seen in this patient. The distinction from heliodermatitis is difficult in many of these patients.

(Figs 2 and 3). As the individual ages, the color tends to deepen with a bluish almost cyanotic color becoming prominent, especially of the nose sometimes referred to as "acrocyanosis" (Fig. 10). The depth and hue of the facial erythema may fluctuate and are influenced by the factors outlined above (Table 1). Close inspection of the skin usually reveals multiple dilated small- to medium-sized blood vessels coursing across the skin surface of the central and lateral cheeks and sometimes along the nose. There may also be a mild degree of facial edema and a slight roughness or scaling on the skin surface and this is some times referred to as "rosacea dermatitis". This roughness is probably related to a defect in the oil content or degree of hydration of the stratum corneum or surface film and possibly explains the susceptibility to stinging irritation of such patients when exposed to minor irritants (5).

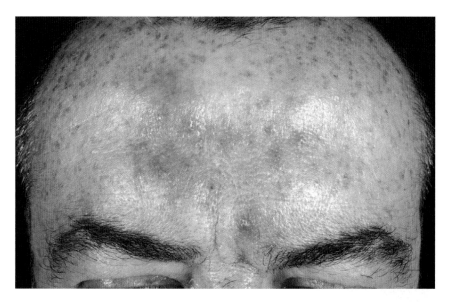

Figure 9 This man has PPR with erythematous papules and pustules on a central facial distribution. His forehead is shown here with heightening of erythema by dilatation of the perilesional blood vessels. Telangiectasias are not a feature of this man's rosacea and the erythema is referred to as being "inflammatory" and likely to settle with treatment of the papulopustular lesions. Much of this erythema cleared following treatment of the inflammatory lesions with topical azelaic acid 15% gel applied twice daily for three weeks.

HISTOPATHOLOGY

In contrast to the very distinctive clinical picture of marked facial erythema, flushing, and telangiectasias, the histopathologic findings in a facial skin biopsy from a patient with ETTR are relatively mild and not diagnostic. The epidermis usually appears normal or slightly atrophic and a mild surface scale may be present. Mid and upper dermal blood vessels usually appear prominent and there may be a mild perivascular infiltrate composed mainly of lymphocytes with an admixture of histeocytes.The most consistent abnormality is a change to the collagen of the upper dermis. This loses its characteristic threadlike morphology and is replaced by an amorphous congealed appearance, so called "solar elastosis" best shown on Periodic Acid Schiff (PAS) staining. This finding, although characteristic of ETTR, is not diagnostic and represents the result of chronic actinic damage.

DIFFERENTIAL DIAGNOSIS AND INVESTIGATIONS

We have already discussed the difficulty in distinguishing between ETTR and chronic photodamage (heliodermatitis). Photosensitive eruptions, either due to topical photosensitizers applied to or coming into contact with the skin of the face

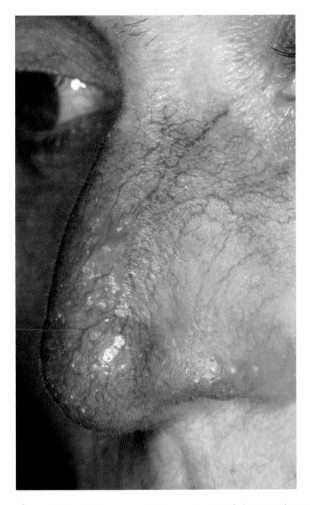

Figure 10 An "acrocyanotic" appearance of the nose is produced in this patient with longstanding ETTR and prominent nasal telangiectatic vessels.

or drugs or disease causing photosensitivity, can mimic ETTR, but an adequate history should identify most of these cases.

Photodistributed telangiectasias mistaken for rosacea have been reported as a side effect of calcium channel–blocking agents. These drugs have vasodilatory actions and are used in the treatment of arterial hypertension (6).

The most important condition to differentiate from ETTR is systemic lupus erythematosus (SLE). The "butterfly rash" of the latter condition (particularly in its early stages or in mild cases) has a similar appearance and distribution to ETTR (Fig. 12), but telangiectasias and flushing are not usually the part of

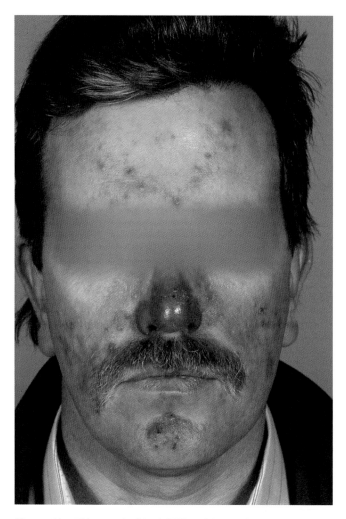

Figure 11 This man had both PPR (with prominent papules and pustules on the fore-head) and ETTR (with persistent erythema and telangiectasias of the nose). The bright red appearance of his nose caused considerable social discomfort.

the clinical picture. However, when the disease is longstanding and particularly if potent topical steroids have been used to treat the cutaneous facial eruption, telangiectasias and persistent facial erythema form part of the clinical picture (Fig. 13). Patients with SLE often have other areas of cutaneous involvement such as the sides and V of the neck. In addition, such individuals are often systemically unwell complaining of symptoms such as tiredness, arthralgias, headaches, etc. Serologic screening for the presence of antinuclear (ANA and anti-DNA) and anticytoplasmic (anti-Ro and anti-La) antibodies should be carried out in cases of

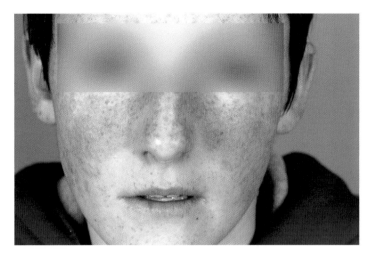

Figure 12 This young woman with systemic lupus erythematosus (SLE) shows the typical "butterfly" distribution of facial erythema extending across the cheeks from the dorsum of the nose. Telangiectasias are not a marked feature of this patient's skin lesions.

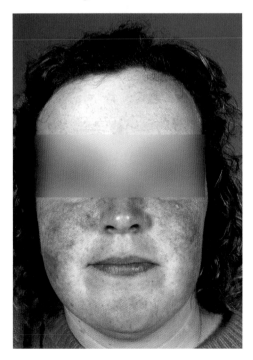

Figure 13 This older patient has longstanding SLE and has used potent topical steroids to control her facial skin lesions. Persistent facial erythema and telangiectasias are prominent, at least partially due to the side effects of her topical therapy.

doubt. Skin biopsy for both histopathologic examination and immunofluoresence can also be helpful, as patients with lupus will show characteristic findings.

Practice Point: The young woman in Figure 12 was referred for investigation and workup. Her astute family doctor had noted the sudden onset of persistent facial erythema after sun exposure combined with profound tiredness, joint pains and loss of energy and had queried the possibility of SLE. Serologic screening showed positive antinuclear antibodies. Systemic steroids were required to control her condition.

Comment: The comprehensive history taken by the family doctor together with the system review pointed to the correct diagnosis.

Patients with dermatomyositis may also present with a facial photosensitive rash similar to SLE. These individuals usually have associated muscle weakness and serology reveals positive anti-Jo antibodies.

Seborrheic dermatitis may sometimes mimic ETTR giving rise to facial erythema, but this is not as intense as that seen in patients with ETTR having a slight yellow to orange tinge to the skin. There is usually a prominent, slightly greasy scale present on the skin surface accentuated at the folds of the nostrils (alae nasi). Atypical distributions can cause problems in making the diagnosis (Fig. 14). Pityriasis capitis (dandruff) is frequently present in individuals with seborrheic dermatitis and in male patients they may be scaling on the central chest, an area unaffected by rosacea. However, it should be recognized that both rosacea and seborrheic dermatitis may both occur simultaneously in the same individual, so that a combination of clinical signs may be seen. It is important to recognize accompanying seborrheic dermatitis in rosacea patients as without treatment of the seborrhoeic element the overall outcome will be less than optimal. Epidermal hyperkeratosis (in which yeast elements may be found) and spongiosis are the typical histologic features of seborrheic dermatitis, but a skin biopsy is rarely required to make this diagnosis.

Facial atopic dermatitis in adult patients or other forms of facial dermatitis, especially in those who have been applying moderate or strong topical steroids to their faces over prolonged periods, can also mimic ETTR. However, there is usually a history of atopy and typically other skin areas are involved.

Disorders of flushing (see chap. 2) can sometimes be confused with ETTR. Careful and accurate clinical history and appropriate investigations should help to differentiate these from ETTR. Contact dermatitis (which may be airborne) or photo contact dermatitis may occasionally cause diagnostic difficulty and require an accurate history as well as patch testing or phototesting to elucidate their cause.

Other rarer conditions that may rarely need to be considered in a patient presenting with features suggestive of ETTR are listed in Table 2. These include erysipelas (see Fig. 1), Jessner's lymphocytic infiltrate, polymorphic light eruption,

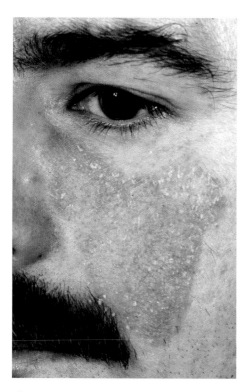

Figure 14   This man has seborrheic dermatitis with an erythematous plaque on the medial cheek. Note the prominent surface scale and the slight orange/yellow hue to the skin lesion. He had in addition a similar plaque on the other cheek and evidence of pityriasis capitis. ETTR is not typically associated with such large adherent scale.

Table 2   Differential Diagnosis of ETTR

Heliodermatitis/atopic dermatitis/contact and photo contact dermatitis
Photodermatitis (including drug-induced
   photodermatitis/telangiectasias)
Disorders of flushing (see chap. 2)
Systemic lupus erythematosus/Dermatomyositis
Seborrheic dermatitis
Topical steroid misuse
Facial Erysipelas/Jessner's lymphocytic infiltrate/polymorphic light
   eruption
Granuloma faciale/lymphocytoma cutis/ facial sarcoid

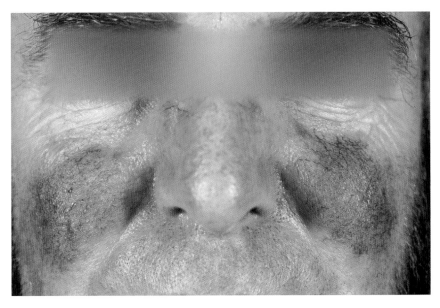

Figure 15 Erythematous plaques with a violaceous hue and surface telangiectatic vessels were the presenting features in this patient. Dioscopy suggested the presence of granulomas and a skin biopsy showed multiple noncaseating granulomas in the skin confirming the diagnosis of cutaneous sarcoid. Pulmonary involvement was demonstrated in the subsequent work-up and he was commenced on systemic steroid therapy with resolution of his skin and lung disease.

lymphocytoma cutis, granuloma faciale, and facial sarcoid. Sarcoid in particular can present unusual patterns in the face with telangiectasias and erythema being prominent features of the eruption (Fig. 15). Although these conditions can at times be difficult to distinguish clinically from ETTR, all have distinctive histopathologic changes in the skin that allow their differentiation from ETTR with a skin biopsy.

MANAGEMENT

ETTR is probably the most difficult of the subtypes of rosacea to treat. The treatment of flushing has been covered in the previous section and will not be repeated here. Suffice to say that avoidance of lifestyle and environmental triggers are especially important for patients with ETTR who have flushing tendencies. The various therapeutic interventions have been covered in Chapter 3. In the general approach to the management of ETTR avoidance of facial contact with abrasive or rough materials is important. In addition, chemical or liquid nitrogen peels should not be used as they are poorly tolerated on the ultrasensitive skin of these patients. Cleansing of the skin is best done by using cool or tepid tap water and a mild nonirritating cleanser. Sponges and bath clothes should be avoided because of their abrasive qualities. Use of bland nonperfumed moisturising creams can be helpful to diminish the scaling and dryness that is sometimes seen in this subtype, and should be applied gently with the finger tips avoiding rubbing or massaging the skin surface. Daily application of a high factor (SPF of 30 or greater) sun-block cream is a vital part of the skin care routine of a patient with ETTR, as ultraviolet light is an identified factor in exacerbating the erythema and telangiectasias in most patients. Sun-block creams containing titanium dioxide and zinc oxide are usually well tolerated and vehicle formulations containing dimethicone and cyclomethicone may be less irritating than others (7). Some individuals prefer to use a moisturiser with incorporated sun-block cream. Topical oxymetazoline has recently been suggested as being effective in reducing facial erythema in patients with rosacea and may be worthwhile in some patients with ETTR (8). If the telangiectatic component of ETTR is significant, then consideration should be given to the use of non ablative laser therapy. There are various different lasers that have been shown to be effective in treating these types of lesions, and it is likely that technological improvements will continue to be made with in this therapeutic modality. The target chromophore in the treatment of vascular lesions is oxyhemoglobin and the surrounding vessel absorbs sufficient energy to be coagulated. Treatment with intense pulsed light therapy and diode lasers have been associated with a diminished tendency to purpura, which can be a disturbing effect of laser therapy, and use of such devices are likely to lead to increased patient compliance because the repeated therapies required to treat these lesions (9).

Cosmetic cover is an important element of the management of both male and female patients with ETTR and can go a long way to lessening the social impact of this condition. Agents with a brilliant green or yellow tint may be effective in reducing the erythema of ETTR, and if possible should be applied gently using a brush rather than using a sponge or cloth to avoid the irritant effect of the latter on sensitive skin (see chap. 8).

Use of a tinted sun block cream can provide a degree of cosmetic cover and reduce the number of topical agents required to apply to the skin.

KEY POINTS

- ETTR is characterised by centrofacial erythema, a tendency to flush frequently, and usually prominent facial telangiectasias.
- ETTR is called Subtype 1 rosacea. This does not imply that it is the first in a sequence of skin changes leading to the other rosacea subtypes.
- Several important conditions need to be considered in the differential diagnosis of ETTR

> - Patients with ETTR have sensitive easily irritated skin. They should keep a record of events, environments, dietary or other elements that flare their skin condition.
> - A high factor sun block cream should be applied to the facial skin daily all year round.
> - Oxymetazoline may diminish facial erythema and non ablative laser therapy coagulate telangiectatic vessels.
> - Seborrhoeic dermatitis may accompany ETTR (and other subtypes of rosacea) and should be treated appropriately in these patients.

REFERENCES

1. Wilkin J, Dahl M, Detmar M, et al. Standard classification of rosacea: Report of the National Rosacea Society Expert Committee on the Classification and Staging of Rosacea. J Am Acad Dermatol 2002; 46: 584–587.
2. Marks R. Concepts in the pathogenesis of rosacea. Brit J Dermatol 1968; 80:170–177.
3. Lavker RM, Kligman AM. Chronic heliodermatitis: A morphologic evaluation of chronic actinic dermal damage with emphasis on the role of mast cells. J Invest Dermatol 1988; 90:325–330.
4. Pons-Guiraud A. Dry skin in dermatology: A complex physiopathology JEADV 2007; 21(suppl 2):1–4.
5. Lonne-Rahm S, Fischer T, Berg M. Stinging and Rosacea. Acta Dermatovener 1999; 79:460–461.
6. Silvester JF, Albares MP, Carnero L, . Photodistributed felodipine-induced facial telangiectasia. J Am Acad Dermatol 2001; 45:323–324.
7. Powell FC. Rosacea. N Eng J Med 2005; 352:793–803.
8. Shanler SD, Ondo AL. Successful treatment of the erythema and flushing of rosacea using a topically applied selective alpha-1adrenergic receptor agonist, oxymetazoline. Arch Dermatol 2007; 143: 1369–1371.
9. Tan R, Tope WP. Pulsed dye Laser therapy of rosacea improves erythema, symptomology, and quality of life. J Amer Acad Dermatol 2004; 51:592–599.

FURTHER READING

Logan RA, and Griffiths WAD. Climatic factors and rosacea. In: Acne and Rosacea. Martin Dunitz Publishers, 1988.
   Comment: A study published in the proceedings of this symposium showed conflicting results of the effects of sunlight on rosacea. The majority of patients with rosacea reported that sunlight was detrimental to their skin condition, but one-third reported improvement. Other interesting reports are contained in this publication.
Marks R. Sun damaged skin. Martin Dunitz Publishers 1992.
   Comment: An interesting and instructive little book looking at the effects of solar radiation on human skin. Shows erythema and telangiectasias as a consequence to lack of support of dermal vessels due to collagen degeneration.

5

Papulopustular (Subtype 2) Rosacea

".... There was a Summoner with us at that Inn,
His face on fire like a cherubim,
For he had carbuncles ....
No quicksilver, lead ointment, tartar creams,
No brimstone, no boric, so it seems,
Could make a salve that had the power to bite,
Clean up or cure his whelks of knobbly white,
Or purge the pimples sitting on his cheeks.
Garlic he loved, and onions too, and leeks,
And drinking strong red wine till all was hazy."

Chaucer, *(Canterbury Tales)*

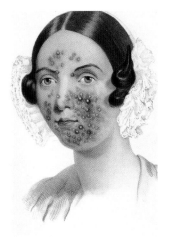

Figure 1 This beautiful drawing illustrates the case of a young woman who appears to have severe "varus gutta rosacea" or couperose as papulopustular subtype 2 rosacea was known on the European continent in the nineteenth century. The differentiation from certain varients of "red acne" can be difficult in some patients.

DEFINITION

Papulopustular rosacea (PPR) is the subtype of rosacea that corresponds most closely to the original concept of rosacea, or "acne rosacea" as was called when the condition was first described in the early 1800s. PPR can be defined as the recurrent eruption of multiple small, nonpainful, dome-shaped, hemispherical, copper- to red-colored papules with less numerous papulopustular lesions (tiny yellow–white fluid collections at the apex of some of the papules). Lesions tend to occur on the centrofacial skin, focusing on the central forehead, dorsum of the nose, medial third of the cheeks (largely avoiding the alae nasi), and the mid-chin areas (Fig. 2).

The inflammatory lesions may be slightly tender and often occur in crops (several papules and pustules appear at the same time or closely following each other in appearance). They last from two to four weeks and without treatment often gradually fade to a pale pink color before flattening and clearing, without leaving any residual scarring. New lesions appear as the older ones fade if effective treatment is not instituted. The condition waxes and wanes, sometimes appearing to go into partial remission, and at other times becoming active and inflammatory for no apparent reason. Some patients complain of recurrent episodes of facial flushing that can predate the appearance of the inflammatory lesions, and preceding fixed facial erythema and/or telangiectasias are present in other patients. However, many individuals with PPR say that their papules and pustules arose without preceding

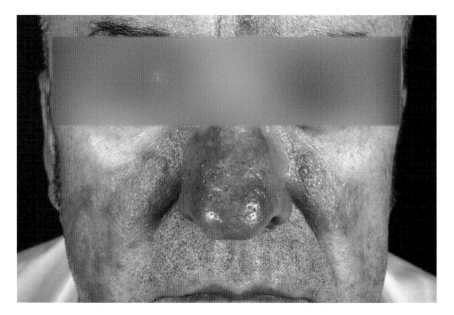

Figure 2   Marked erythema of the nose and medial cheeks with inflammatory papules surmounting the nose in a middle-aged man with PPR. The central forehead and chin were also affected in this patient who was actuely self conscious of his facial appearance. He responded well to metronidazole 0.7% cream applied twice daily over a period of 4 weeks with complete clearing of his inflammatory lesions and a lessening of facial erythema.

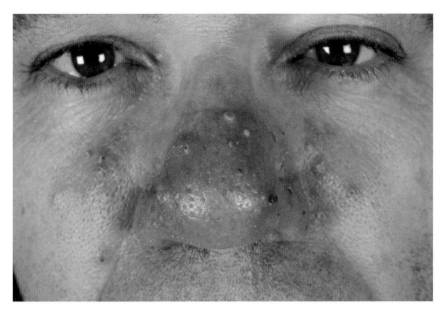

Figure 3 Erythema, prominent follicular openings, papules, and large pustules on the nose are the main features of this man's PPR. Note the erythema extending on the medial cheeks with scattered papules on the skin surface. Telangiectasias are not a feature of this man's PPR and he did not complain of preceding flushing.

events on skin that they assumed had been normal up to that point. There may be related ocular symptoms or inflammatory changes of ocular rosacea (OR) in as many as 50% of patients with PPR (1).

DISTRIBUTION

The distribution of the inflammatory lesions in subtype 2 rosacea is characteristically on the centrofacial skin involving the dorsal aspect of the nose and the medial cheeks, often with relative sparing the alae nasi (Fig. 3).

Practice Point: There is a major cosmetic impact when the nose is involved with PPR as shown in this patient (Fig. 3). He had applied a sulfur-containing cream, but it irritated his skin and he was unable to continue therapy. Treatment with minocycline 100 mg daily was initiated and three weeks later the inflammation had dimished markedly. Azelaic acid gel (15%) applied twice daily was then added with complete control and minocin was discontinued.

Comment: In patients with severe PPR, topical therapies can irritate inflamed skin. Systemic treatment may be required initially to "calm" the skin sufficiently to tolerate the topical agent.

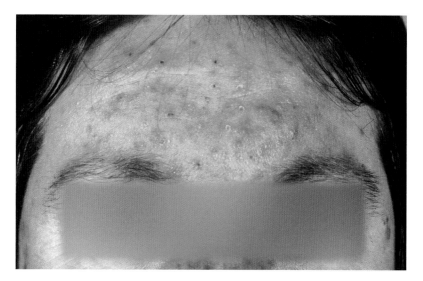

Figure 4 Involvement of the central forehead is a characteristic feature of patients with moderate to severe PPR. The skin of the lateral forehead appears normal in color and there are no inflammatory lesions in these areas.

The center of the forehead is similarly favored by the inflammatory lesions, which are often grouped together (Fig. 4). Lesions can occur sporadically on the more lateral cheeks and in severe cases can be numerous in this location even extending on to the sides of the neck (Fig. 5). In some patients with male pattern baldness, the eruption of papules and pustules may extend onto the bald scalp in continuity with the facial eruption (Fig. 6).

> **Practice Point:** The patient shown in Figure 6 was referred for treatment of scalp "folliculitis." Examination revealed typical PPR of the face and early rhinophyma. Treatment with doxycycline was initiated and the lesions cleared. His skin and scalp remained clear with topical metronidazole 0.75% gel applied twice daily which has been continued to date.
> *Comment: Rosacea of the scalp in patients with male pattern alopecia is not uncommon and suggests that the miniaturized follicles have become susceptible in some way to inflammation as involvement of follicles with terminal hairs (i.e. the hairs growing on the normal scalp) is not usually seen. Systemic therapy is typically required to get a rapid response to extensive cutaneous involvement of PPR as in this case. Topical therapy is usually sufficient to maintain the remission once this has been achieved. The choice of which formulation of topical agent to prescribe depends on the likely tolerance by the patient. Some patients find gel preparations cause a stinging sensation and so prefer creams. Others with less sensitive skin like gel formulations. The patient will often express their preference if asked.*

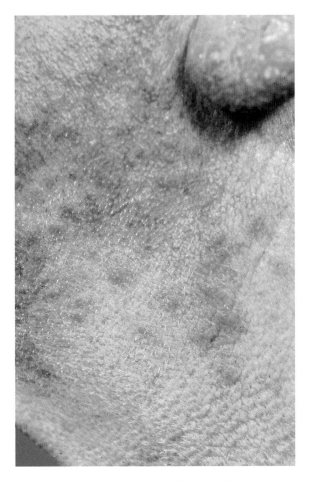

Figure 5   In severe or extensive PPR, the typical erythematous papules and some pustules can extend to the sides of the neck as shown in this patient who had severe disease. Note also the involvement of the lobe of the ear.

In patients who have extensive facial involvement with PPR grouped pustules on a background erythema may be seen on the superior aspect of the helix of the ears as shown in Figure 7(A). After appropriate treatment these inflammatory lesions can resolve without residua, Figure 7(B). Typically the eruption of PPR affects both sides of the face in a symmetrical fashion, but occasionally lesions may be limited in their distribution with involvement primarily of one side of the face. Such a distribution should raise the possibility of tinea faciei as an alternative diagnosis and prompt appropriate investigations (see differential diagnosis). A concentration of the papules and pustules in clusters around the eyes or mouth should alert the clinician to the possible diagnosis of periocular or perioral dermatitis (2). Although extra-facial papules and pustules of rosacea have

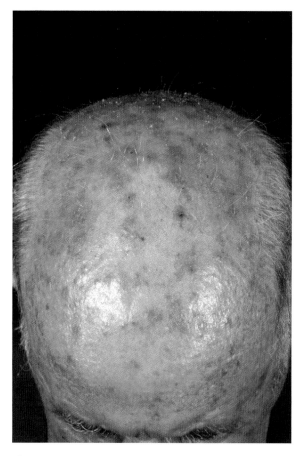

Figure 6 Involvement of the bald scalp with papules and pustules in continuity with the lesions on the face is regularly seen in patients with male pattern alopecia and PPR. With normal hair growth, scalp involvement is not a feature of rosacea.

been described, mainly on the trunk and abdomen (3), in the author's opinion, it is impossible to distinguish between the inflammatory lesions described in these reports of "extra facial rosacea" from the much commoner folliculitis, which has a predilection for these areas.

BACKGROUND

PPR occupies the central point in the spectrum of cutaneous changes that are classified under the encompassing title of "rosacea." Apart from rhinophyma, PPR is the most easily recognized subtype of rosacea. Therapeutic efficacy of new pharmaceutical products for rosacea are usually assessed by carrying out "lesion counts" (i.e., counting the numbers of papules and pustules) before, during, and

(A)   (B)

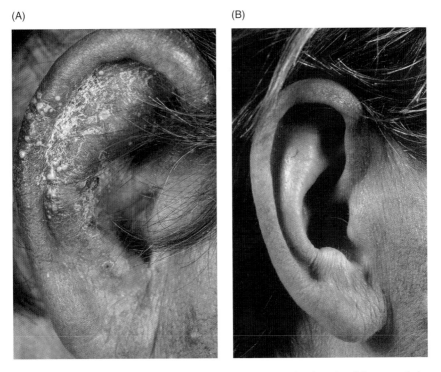

Figure 7 (**A**) This patient who had severe extensive PPR developed striking pustulation of the helix of the ears. Auricular involvement (most often of the ear lobes) to a mild degree is occasionally seen in patients with less severe PPR. (**B**) Following systemic treatment (minocycline 100 mgs daily for 6 weeks was prescribed in this patient's case) the pustules cleared completely without any residual scarring or postinflammatory pigmentation.

after treatment as well as measuring the degree of facial erythema at these times. PPR is, paradoxically, the easiest type of rosacea to treat, with the inflammatory papules and pustules often responding readily to topical or systemic therapies (often antibiotics) or combinations of these modalities. The background erythema diminishes with these therapies but usually does not fully clear.

The etiology of this PPR, as with all other subtypes of rosacea, is unknown. However many different etiological theories have been proposed.

> *"His rosy cheeks showed that he had good health. His fleshiness, which was not too apparent, showed that he had a good appetite, and the reddish tinge in his nose and the pimple on the tip of it, showed according to his enemies that he was a 'little fond of the bottle'."*
>
> Liam O'Flaherty, *Thy Neighbours Wife*

In the early descriptions of the disorder it was postulated that dietary factors (excessive intake of meats, highly seasoned foods, pastries, or sweets), hot meals or liquids (soup, tea, or coffee), and especially alcohol were considered important in provoking the eruption.

In women, "menstrual problems" and "psychological upset" were thought to contribute to the onset of the problem. Gastrointestinal disturbances, "functional or organic," were thought to cause exacerbation of rosacea in both sexes, with supplementary hydrochloric acid (to be taken before meals) and pepsin often prescribed for suffers. Constipation was also blamed for producing a build up of "toxic factors" which then provoked the eruption of papules and pustules.

> *"Improper assimilation of food and lessened elimination through constipation produce toxic substances are factors . . ."*
> Ormsby and Montgomery, *Textbook of Dermatology (1947)*

Measures these medical experts advised in the 1940s included, remaining in the bed for breakfast (to induce relaxation), slow eating of meals (to avoid flushing), taking hydrochloric acid supplements with meals (to correct hypochlorhydria), reducing the intake of carbohydrates (because of intestinal intolerance), increasing the quantity of meat intake (to provide more protein and stimulate hydrochloric acid production in the stomach), increasing the intake of butter fat (to combat the reduction in weight seen in the "thin, intense rosacea patient"), and taking laxatives (to correction of constipation).

Another theory suggested that frequent and prolonged episodes of flushing eventually lead to the development of fixed, dilated (telangiectatic) blood vessels in the face. These widened blood vessels resulted in "stagnation" of blood flow and leakage of "serum and other materials" into the dermis. Inflammatory changes (papules and pustules) were postulated to develop subsequent to the host's defensive reactive mechanisms. However, as we have seen earlier (chapter 2), this theory did not satisfactorily explain the sequence of evolution of the disorder in many patients.

Some researchers studying the reactivity of the facial blood vessels suggested that there was a defect in central thermostatic sensors at the brain level, with faulty temperature monitoring leading to persistent facial vasodilatation in an effort to correct apparently elevated central brain–blood temperature (6). The concurrence of PPR in patients with the carcinoid syndrome seemed to validate the hypothesis that inflammatory lesions develop consequent to frequent and prolonged flushing. However, these case reports are so rare that they probably represent the chance concurrence of two disorders (one fairly common and one rare) in one individual. Even large published series of patients with the carcinoid syndrome do not record any consistent finding of facial rosacea and it is not generally regarded as a likely finding in patients with longstanding disease.

In keeping with the early suggestions that the cause of rosacea may lie within the gastrointestinal tract, some recent investigators have suggested that *Helicobacter pylori* infection of the stomach might be incriminated in provoking

PPR. The suggested pathogenesis involves release of gastrin and possibly other hormonal mediators from the gastrointestinal tract. It is postulated that these subsequently have a systemic effect leading to frequent facial flushing and then persistent vasodilatation and telangiectasias on the face. However, several studies from different countries have failed to validate this hypothesis (7).

Another theory of pathogenesis relates to the presence of abundant *Demodex folliculorum* mites in the facial skin of patients with rosacea. These small worm-like organisms are inhabitants of the sebaceous follicles of normal adult facial skin. They were first described in the 1800s, but their role in the homeostasis of facial skin is unknown. They have been reported to transport bacteria on the skin surface, and their population can increase markedly in certain circumstances (see below). They can be easily extracted from the follicles where they are found, often in groups, head downward, feeding on sebaceous material. They have eight short stubby legs with claw-like end processes (Fig. 8A and B), which they use to move about the facial skin surface from one follicle to another. This apparently occurs at night (it has been shown that the mites react negatively to light.) These organisms seem to live in a harmonious relationship with their hosts and in normal circumstances do not excite an inflammatory reaction in the skin. It is not known if they perform any useful function in human skin, and it is probably impossible to fully eradicate them as the skin seems to become recolonized rapidly following antimite treatment. In patients with rosacea, these mites are

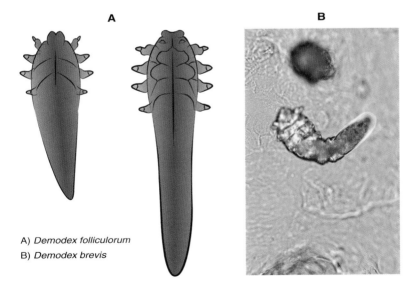

A   **B**

A) *Demodex folliculorum*
B) *Demodex brevis*

Figure 8   (A) This diagram shows the worm-like bodies of *Demodex folliculorum* (which lives in the pilosebaceous canal) and *Demodex brevis* (which lives in the sebaceous glands). In spite of their ubiquitous presence in healthy human adults, little is known of the life cycle of these interesting and complex organisms. (B) A mite extracted from the facial skin of a patient with rosacea using the skin surface biopsy technique showing its ventral surface.

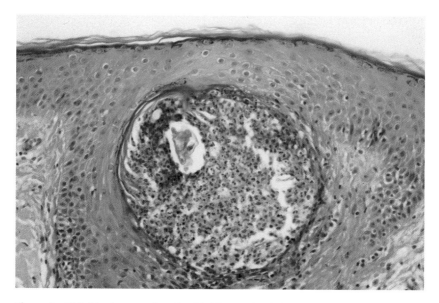

Figure 9 This histology section of a skin biopsy of an inflammatory papule from a patient with rosacea. This shows the upper portion of a follicular canal with the head of a demodex mite surrounded by a collection inflammatory cells (neutrophils). The overlying epidermis appears normal.

greatly increased in number and are found mainly in the centrofacial convexities—the areas typically affected by the inflammatory papules and pustules. Histologic sections of inflammatory lesions show the pathologic changes to be centered on the follicles and mites or the fragments of disrupted mites are often seen in the follicular canals surrounded by inflammatory cells (Fig. 9). Sometimes ruptured follicles are seen with particles of demodex mites extruded into the dermis. In these cases foreign body granuloma formation to the follicular keratin and/or the mite is a feature of the histopathologic changes. Immunosuppressed patients (with HIV infection or on immunosuppressive therapy or patients having renal dialysis) or those who have applied immune-modulating drugs (topical steroids/calcineurin inhibitors) to the face may also have increased numbers of demodex mites on the skin. This suggests a possible role of local immune mechanisms restricting the demodex population in normal facial skin. Some immunosuppressed patients may also develop a pustular eruption similar to rosacea with multiple mites identified not only on skin biopsies, but also visualized by microscopic examination of scale obtained by gently scraping the skin surface. In some individuals these eruptions were cleared when antimite treatment was used. Finally, it has been shown that these mites have related bacteria, some of which are susceptible to the antibiotics used to treat the papules and pustules of rosacea. These facts could explain the effectiveness of topical and systemic antibiotics in the management of this disorder

(8). Another recent finding which may have relevance to our understanding of PPR is the discovery that antimicrobial peptide (AMP) production and/or metabolism appears to be altered in patients with rosacea. These peptides or related enzymes can produce inflammatory lesions similar to the papules and pustules of PPR when injected into the skin of the mouse model. Vitamin D also has an influence on AMP production and may provide a link with ultraviolet light and inflammatory lesions in patients with rosacea. It may be that a synthesis of these new areas of knowledge will provide insight into the causation of PPR in the future.

CLINICAL FEATURES

PPR is easily recognized in its typical form by the presence of multiple (usually greater than 5), small (2 to 3 mm), bright erythematous papules which may be in various stages of evolution. These inflammatory lesions arise on the central facial convexities, i.e., the dorsum of the middle and distal nose, the proximal cheeks and cheekbones (but usually not at the alae nasi), as well as the central forehead and sometimes the middle area of the chin. As already mentioned. the eruption is usually symmetrical and some papules (usually the minority) have a surmounting focus of pustulation covering the upper third of the dome-shaped papule (Fig. 10).

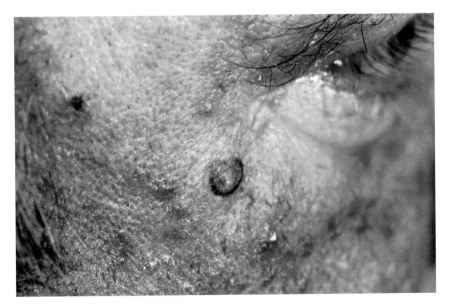

Figure 10   This closeup view shows the surface pustulation (circled) of an inflammatory papule on the cheek of a patient who had severe PPR. In this patients case, the eruption extended to the lateral cheeks. Note the relative sparing of the skin in the infraorbital region where the uninvolved skin appears pale by comparison with the erythema of the affected skin.

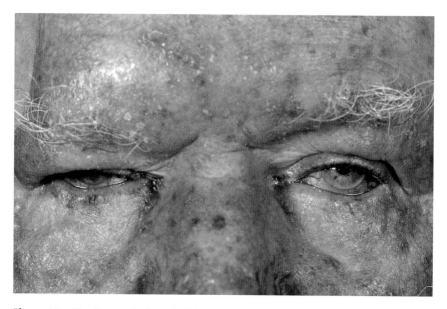

Figure 11 The degree of edema in this man's skin is demonstrated by the partial closure of his right eye. Facial erythema, scaling papules, pustules and conjunctival injection were the other features of this patient's facial skin who had severe PPR with accompanying moderate ocular rosacea (OR).

Some papules and pustules are the central focus of tiny radiating telangiectatic vessels that heighten the appearance of erythema. Occasionally, patients may develop papules and pustules on a background of persistent facial erythema, some telangiectasias, and a tendency to frequent flushing (ETTR). In other patients, there is evidence of "rosacea dermatitis" with erythema, scaling, and inflammation in the distribution of the inflammatory lesions. The combination of the above features in a patient with fully developed PPR gives a striking clinical picture of vivid erythema, scaling, papules and pustules, and edema (Fig. 11). This edema is reactive to the intense cutaneous inflammation and typically reduces but often not fully subsides after its successful treatment (usually requiring systemic antibiotic therapy). Such secondary edema should be distinguished from the diffuse idiopathic solid upper facial edema (sometimes called Morbihan disease or Edematous Rosacea). Morbihan disease (named after a region of northern France were patients with this problem were first identified) typically is not preceded by significant cutaneous inflammation (Fig. 12). The cause of this type of facial swelling is unknown, and any relationship of Morbihan disease to the subtypes of rosacea described here is doubtful.

The severity of PPR may be graded according to the numbers of papules and pustules (few, several, or many) and whether plaques (confluent

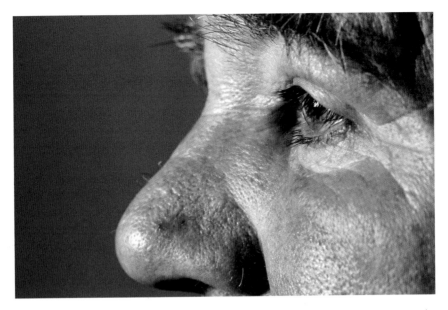

Figure 12 The facial edema of Morbihan disease can be difficult to demonstrate in a photograph. This man had firm erythematous nonpitting, nonpainful swelling of the upper face without preceding inflammatory lesions. The edema can best be appreciated here as a swelling of the skin below the eye and an exaggerated skin fold at the inner canthus of the eye.

inflammatory lesions on a raised area of erythema) are present as shown in Figure 13.

DIFFERENTIAL DIAGNOSIS AND INVESTIGATIONS

Rosaceiform dermatitis is a recently introduced term used to describe the abrupt onset of facial erythema and stinging with small papules and numerous pustules erupting in the distribution of application of calcineurin inhibitors. Rosaceiform dermatitis may be induced in patients who may or may not have a previous history of rosacea (9). Topical calcineurin inhibitors are sometimes prescribed for patients who have seborrheic dermatitis or atopic dermatitis of the face. They act as topical immunomodulators and inhibit T-cell activation and thus may reduce the host inflammatory response. *D. folliculorum* mites (see above) are found in abundance in some individuals affected with this disorder, and their proliferation may be facilitated by the reduced level of immune reactivity.

An eruption similar to rosaceiform dermatitis can be seen in persons who have applied potent topical steroid creams to their faces over prolonged periods and is referred to as "steroid induced rosacea–like dermatitis" (Fig. 14).

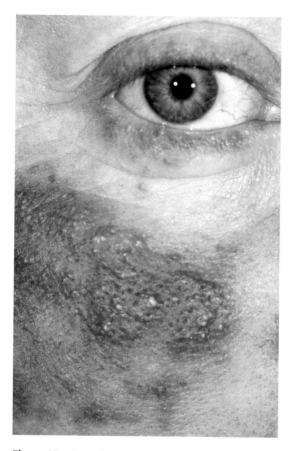

Figure 13   A confluent erythematous plaque studded with surface pustulation is a feature of severe PPR as seen in this patient. Note the ocular involvement as evidenced by the inflammatory lesions on his lower lid. (Reproduced with permission from ref 14).

Practice Point: The young woman whose face is shown in Fig 14 had been applying a potent cortisone cream to her face for several months. When she tried to discontinue its use, her skin flared severely. Her face became progressively red and the skin appeared thinned and bruised easily. She began to develop red spots on the affected skin and was referred for treatment of "rosacea".

Comment: The facial skin of some individuals seems to get "hooked" on topical cortisone creams. The solution is to continue with the use of a weaker strength cortisone for a short period until it can be stopped completely. This "weaning" process was successful in the patient shown here and was combined with oxytetracycline 500 mg twice daily over two months. Stopping the topical steroid abruptly will result in a "withdrawl crisis" and the patient will either revert to her strong cortisone cream or change physicians.

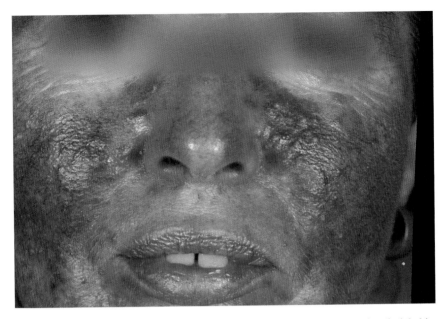

Figure 14 This lady had applied a potent topical corticosteroid cream to her facial skin for prolonged periods. Note the intense erythema, atrophy of the skin, and striking telangiectasias. Scattered papules are visible (mainly on the medial cheek areas) giving the patient a "rosaceiform" appearance.

These patients have also been shown to have a major increase in the demodex mite count on their facial skin using the cyanoacrylate skin biopsy technique (10). The relationship of the eruptions induced by application of cortisone creams to the skin and PPR is unclear. They serve as interesting disease models and suggest that altering the cutaneous immune response in the face may permit local ecologic changes in the follicular canal. This could result in the facial demodex population flourishing, which in turn may result in the genesis of inflammatory lesions.

Acne vulgaris can be easily differentiated from PPR in the majority of cases. Patients with acne vulgaris have generally a younger age of onset of disease, have much less facial erythema, and have oily, greasy skin with large pores, some of which have open comedones (blackheads) or closed comedones (whiteheads). Large cystic lesions and scarring are features of acne vulgaris as is the involvement of the upper back and anterior chest. Although comedones (blackheads or whiteheads) are not features usually seen in rosacea and monomorphic lesions are uncommon in acne vulgaris, there are patients in whom the differentiation between these two common facial dermatoses may prove problematic (Fig. 15). Patients who have had acne vulgaris as teenagers and subsequently develop PPR may have residual scarring and comedones from the acne vulgaris, which forms the background for the eruption of the papules and pustules of rosacea. Some older patients who have otherwise typical acne vulgaris develop quite marked facial

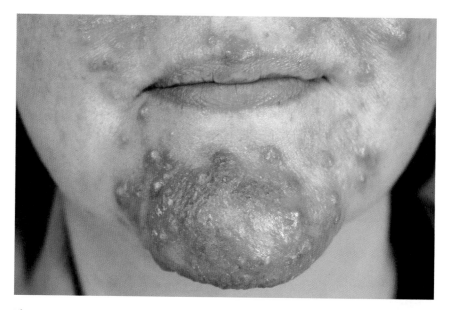

Figure 15 This young woman has large coalescing inflammatory lesions with marked erythema on her chin, medial cheeks and central forehead. The distribution and erythema suggested the diagnosis of rosacea, while the deep inflammatory nature of the lesions were more typical of acne vulgaris. She was treated with low dose isotretinoin and her skin lesions settled.

erythema, which can be difficult to distinguish from PPR, while other patients (usually male) with typical PPR have oily skin with prominent pores suggestive of the acne vulgaris sufferer (Fig. 16). Some female patients can have a rapid onset of multiple inflammatory cystic facial lesions with marked erythema and a tendency to scarring. The nosology of this group of patients has been discussed in Chapter 3. Terms such as "rosacea conglobata," "rosacea fulminans," and "pyoderma faciale" (an acne vulgaris variant) have been used to describe these eruptions. This latter viewpoint would seem more likely, as little of the clinical presentation (apart from the facial erythema) resembles rosacea, while the deep inflammation of the cystic lesions and the tendency to scarring are hallmarks of acne vulgaris.

Perioral dermatitis can usually be distinguished from PPR by its distribution on the face and the morphology of the skin lesions. As the name implies, the typical distribution of this eruption of fine vesicles, pustules, and papules is in a symmetrical fashion encircling the mouth with a zone of normal skin separating the eruption from the vermillion border of the lips (Figure 17). Sometimes the eruption can occur around the eyes when the term periocular dermatitis is used, and lesions can occur in the perinasal region. Occasionally the vesicles, papules, and pustules may be distributed in an asymmetrical fashion. Smaller and more superficial than the papules and pustules of PPR, the lesions, (firm erythematous

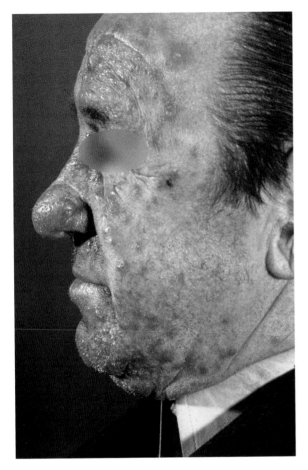

Figure 16 It can be difficult to distinguish between acne vulgaris (with erythema) and PPR (with seborrhoea) in some older male patients. The central distribution of inflammatory lesions and the presence of early rhinophyma were helpful indicators of PPR in this man. Treatment with oxytetracycline 500 mgs twice daily combined with topical metronidazole gel lead to a marked improvement of his skin appearance.

papules, papulovesicles, and papulopustules), are often grouped ("agminated"). They are typically all in the same stage of evolution, in contrast to the inflammatory lesions of PPR that may be more variable in their stages of development. Erythema and scaling are two other constant findings, and the patient often complains of intolerance to sunlight and to local applications (including cosmetics and hot water). It is thought that bacterial or yeast overgrowth may give rise to the inflammatory lesions in patients with perioral dermatitis. Patients (females are most often affected) often give a history of having used topical corticosteroid creams before the onset of the eruption. Occasionally inhaled corticosteroids are responsible for

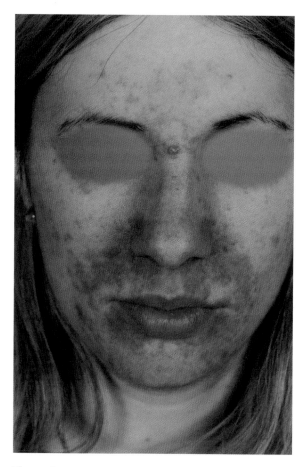

Figure 17 Perioral dermatitis is evident in this young woman who had previously applied a mild topical steroid cream repeatedly over several weeks to her face. The erythema is striking, as is the distribution around the mouth but avoiding the vermillion border of the lips. Discontinuation of the topical steroid and a six-week course of minocycline 100 mgs daily cleared her eruption. Her skin showed no sign of relapse with a follow-up of 6 months.

this eruption (11). Discontinuation of the use of the topical corticosteroid and a systemic antibiotic (tetracyclines, minocycline, or erythromycin) taken over a six-week period usually results in a complete clearance of the eruption. Subsequent relapse of perioral dermatitis is uncommon when the treatment is discontinued (unlike PPR when such relapse is frequent). It should be remembered, that the lesions of PPR may occur in a perioral distribution as shown in Figure 18(A) and a periocular distribution as shown in Figure 18(B). The papules in patients with PPR are usually larger than those seen in perioral dermatitis and vesiculation is not a feature.

(A)

(B)

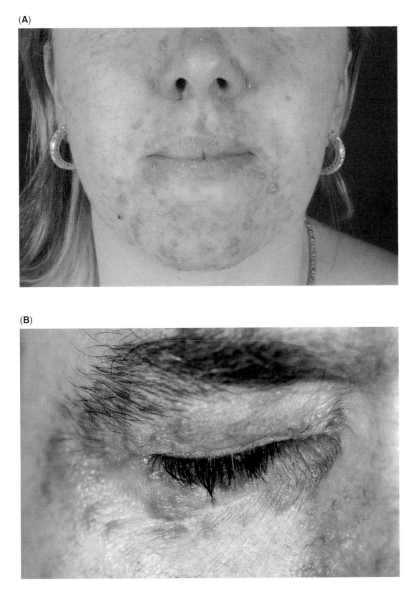

Figure 18 (**A**) Sometimes PPR can occur mainly in a perioral distribution. Usually there are lesions elsewhere as seen on the cheeks and nose of this patient. The papules of PPR are somewhat larger than seen in perioral dermatitis, and the monomorphic appearance is lacking. (**B**) Grouped erythematous papules in various stages of evolution are shown distributed around the eyes in this patient with PPR.

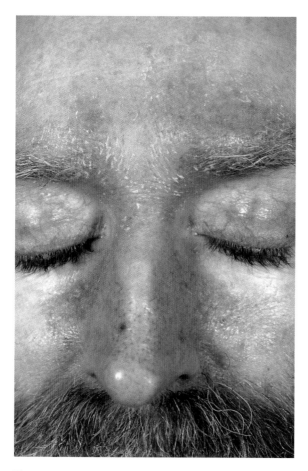

Figure 19   In the majority of cases, the diagnosis of seborrheic dermatitis is made on the distinctive yellow/orange hue of the skin eruption and the typical distribution as seen in this patient. An atypical distribution or the combined picture of PPR, seborrheic dermatitis, and rosacea dermatitis can occasionally give rise to confusion in individual patients.

Seborrheic dermatitis has already been mentioned as a disorder that commonly accompanies PPR. It is important to recognize the features of this eruption, as appropriate therapy should be directed to its treatment or the overall clinical improvement will be suboptimal (see chapter 4). The characteristic greasy yellowish adherent scale closely applied to the alae nasi and eyebrows (Fig. 19), its presence behind the ears and occasionally on the central anterior chest of male patients, together with pityriasis capitis (dandruff) makes the diagnosis straightforward in the typical case.

Pityriasis folliculorum is an often-overlooked clinical entity (12). Patients with this eruption are most frequently female. There is usually a history of rarely

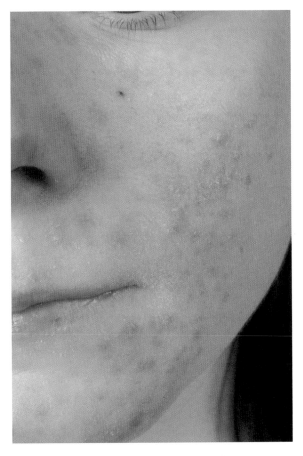

Figure 20 This young woman had not used soap or water on her face for several years. She constantly used moisturisers and cleansing creams to treat her skin. The scattered small erythematous papules are characteristic of pityriasis folliculorum, as is the slightly adherent surface scale. Scraping of the skin surface revealed numerous demodex mites. Her skin cleared with a change of facial skin treatment routine and the application of a sodium sulfacetamide/sulphur cream at night.

using soap or water to cleanse their facial skin but instead using cleansing creams. In addition, these individuals often apply a moisturizing cream twice daily to their facial skin. The skin of the central face and cheeks develops a glistening, slightly roughened surface scaling that has been described as having a "frosty" or "nutmeg grater" appearance caused by follicular plugging by fine white scales. There may be inflammatory lesions (papules and pustules) similar to those seen in rosacea but usually slightly smaller and not as strikingly erythematous (Fig. 20). The patient may complain of a burning or itchy sensation in their facial skin. The diagnosis of pityriasis folliculorum is facilitated by the use of dermatoscopy, which shows a

Table 1   Differential Diagnosis of PPR

Rosaceiform dermatitis (check drug history)
Acne vulgaris (comedones/cysts/scarring/chest and back in males)
Perioral dermatitis (check topical steroid usage)
Seborrheic dermatitis (pityriasis capitis often marked)
Pityriasis folliculorum/demodecosis (skin scraping helpful)
Tinea faceii/Candida (scrapings/swabs for culture)/contact dermatitis
    (patch testing helpful)
Ulerythema ophrogenes/Jessner's lymphocytic infiltrate/lymphocytoma cutis/sarcoid
    (skin biopsy helpful)
Morbihan disease/polycythemia/polymorphic light eruption/photosensitive eruption
    (blood tests/phototesting helpful)

---

distinctive picture of the presence of multiple white keratotic material consisting of keratin encrusted demodex mites protruding upwards from the follicular orifices. Scraping the skin surface with the blunt side of a scalpel blade and spreading the scrapings on a glass slide reveals the presence of multiple dead and living *D. folliculorum* mites. The condition appears to be caused by an overpopulation of mites facilitated by the frequent use of creams and the lack of face washing with soap and water. Resumption of facial washing and a discontinuation of the daily moisturizing regimen are necessary to help clear this condition. More persistent cases of pityriasis folliculorum may require the use of a compound sulphur ointment, antimite treatment, or occasionally systemic antibiotic therapy as outlined above for perioral dermatitis.

Tinea faciei can occasionally be confused with PPR, especially if inadvertently treated with topical steroids. The dermatophytic eruption may be characterized by facial erythema and papules and pustules, but is rarely symmetrical unlike the distribution in most patients with PPR. A well-defined border with a distinctive peripheral scale is often visible to the careful examiner. Skin scrapings for microscopy and fungal culture will establish the diagnosis and topical and/or systemic antifungal therapy will lead to its clearance.

Occasionally, the asymmetry of the facial eruption may be caused by other dermatoses, such as cutaneous sarcoid (Fig. 21). Although sarcoid often mimics other skin conditions, pustules are not a usual feature. A skin biopsy may be required to establish the diagnosis. Other rare disorders that might be considered in the differential diagnosis of unusual presentations of PPR are shown in Table 1.

There is no laboratory test or investigation that will confirm the diagnosis of PPR. Specific investigations may be required to rule out similar appearing conditions (many of which will be identified by listening carefully to the patient's medical history and examining the skin lesions). These include skin swabs for bacterial culture, skin scrapings for the presence of demodex mites, scrapings for fungal KOH and fungal culture, skin biopsy for histologic examination, (and

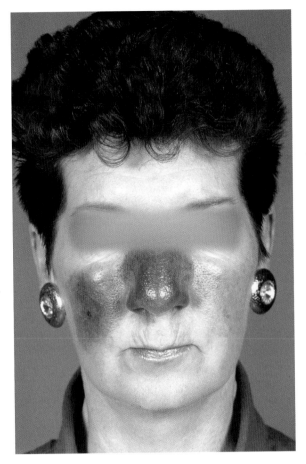

Figure 21 Cutaneous sarcoid is a great mimicker of other dermatoses. The bright facial erythema of this patients face may initially suggest rosacea, but the asymmetry of the eruption, the plaque-like morphology, and dioscopy showing "apple-jelly" nodules will help to establish the clinical diagnosis that is confirmed by finding non caseating dermal granulomas on the skin biopsy.

rarely culture) skin surface biopsy for demodex mite quantification, patch tests, photopatch tests, and very rarely systemic workup with appropriate blood tests and radiological examinations.

MANAGEMENT

PPR is probably the easiest of the rosacea subtypes to manage. Patients are often pleased with the rapid response of the skin lesions to therapy and the lack of residual scarring. However, a comprehensive approach is needed and it is important to consider every element of the patient's eruption and ensure that treatment is adapted accordingly or the clinical response will not be optimal.

The general measures (avoiding irritating substances on the affected skin, applying high factor sun-block creams, appropriate cosmetic cover, and skin cleansing/moisturizing routines) as outlined for patients with ETTR (see chapter 4) also apply to patients who develop PPR. It is well worthwhile spending time explaining the need for these approaches on the patient's first visit, as the effect of this advice if followed is likely to help prolong remissions. Alternatively, failure to address these aspects of the therapy may result in a less-than-satisfactory response to whatever medical therapy is instituted or rapid relapse when treatment is discontinued.

Stress is often identified by patients with PPR as being a factor that causes flares or exacerbations of their skin condition. This element must not be overlooked by the practitioner and appropriate questions asked and advice given regarding stress management or counseling if necessary. Facial massage (for the edematous component of PPR), hypnotherapy and meditation have been suggested as being useful in the management of PPR but proof of efficacy is lacking.

Since herbal treatments for rosacea and other skin conditions are increasingly popular with patients, the practitioner must directly question the individuals with PPR about their usage of these remedies. Many patients will not otherwise volunteer this information (13). While some herbal treatments may indeed prove to be helpful in the management of PPR, the scientific proof of their efficacy is lacking and in the past some herbal preparations have been shown to contain cortisone (which can destabilize rosacea or produce rosaceiform eruptions as we have discussed). There is also the potential for drug interactions if the patient continues to take both prescribed medications and the herbal preparation.

If flushing is a feature of the patient's clinical picture then avoidance of the agents likely to precipitate flushing is important (see chapter 2), and patients should be advised to keep a diary of events so that they can identify the particular agents that tend to cause an exacerbation of the flushing aspect of their PPR.

As indicated in the section on etiology, dietary measures were considered important in the management of PPR by earlier dermatologists. Other than avoiding the dietary precipitants of flushing, there is no reliable evidence to validate dietary measures in the treatment of an individual with PPR. Investigations of possible gastrointestinal abnormalities, including *H. pylori* infection, in these patients is unwarranted unless there are specific clinical indications. Trichloracetic or salicylic acid peels have been reported to be helpful in some patients, but are likely to cause irritation and are best avoided.

The inflammatory papules and pustules of PPR usually respond readily to a variety of topical and systemic agents, mostly antibiotics. Patients should be reminded, however, that telangiectasias and phymatous changes are unlikely to be affected by these treatments.

Mild to moderate PPR will respond well to topical therapy. The range of topical measures used to treat PPR are shown in Table 2. The most frequently used are the various preparations of metronidazole (creams, gels and lotions which may

Table 2   Topical Treatments for PPR

Sodium sulfacetamide/sulfur cleansers
Metronidazole cream/gel/lotion
Azelaic acid cream/gel
Sodium sulfacetamide/sulphur (cream/lotion/cleanser)
Erythromycin solution/gel
Clindamycin lotion/gel Topical benzoyl peroxidea (useful in
    patients with oily skin)
Erythromycin/benzoyl peroxide gel
Clindamycin/benzoyl peroxide gel
Tretinoin cream/lotion/gel Ivermectin cream
Adapalene gel
Retinaldehyde cream
Precipitated sulfur cream ($\pm$ 1% hydrocortisone)
Sulfur/salicylic acid a (cream varying strengths)
Oxymetazolinea (useful for persistent erythema)
Permethrin
Ivermectin

be available in different strengths) and azelaic acid gel. Azelaic acid gel (15%) and the metronidazole preparations are effective treatments when applied twice daily to the skin. Both of these preparations should be applied to the area of skin affected and not solely to inflammatory lesions. An occasional patient will experience an initial burning sensation with azelaic acid, but this usually settles with continued use. When the rosacea clears, treatment should be continued to maintain remission. If the skin remains in remission over several months, the patient can gradually discontinue treatment, initially applying the preparation once daily for two weeks and then on alternate days for two weeks before stopping. If a flare occurs, the patient should reintroduce therapy at the original frequency themselves. In this way, the individual can take over the management of their skin condition with occasional supervision by the physician. Metronidazole 0.75% cream preparation is particularly well tolerated by patients with sensitive skin. In comparative studies it would appear that there is little difference in the efficacy of these products (azelaic acid and metronidazole) and that both are well tolerated. They are particularly effective in clearing the inflammatory lesions of PPR. The erythema may respond better to the azelaic acid preparation, but can be expected to diminish progressively (over several months) following sucessful with either treatment. Topical metronidazole products should not be prescribed to pregnant or lactating females. Experience with the use of azelaic acid by pregnant mothers is too limited to permit assessment of the safety of its used during pregnancy. 10% sodium sulfacetamide and 5% sulfur cream or lotion are also effective topical therapies of PPR and can be used to treat concomitant seborrheic dermatitis. It can also be helpful to treat patients with pityriasis folliculorum as discussed earlier. It should be avoided in patients with sensitivity to sulfur or sulphonamides. Tinted and sunscreen containing preparations of these products are available, which appeal to some patients.

The choice among these topical agents can be difficult. In my opinion, individual patients vary in their tolerance and response to treatment. I usually start my patients with a metronidazole cream or azelaic acid gel applied twice daily. Occasionally the response will be disappointing and this requires the physician to switch from one topical therapy to another to achieve optimal results. I advise my patients that my initial prescription is likely to be successful, but that a follow-up visit is required after three weeks to ensure that they have had a good response. I explain that what works for one patient may not always suit another, but that there is a selection of good treatments available. It is advisable that the physician becomes familiar with the tolerability of two or three topical agents on dry, normal, sensitive and oily skin as well as in patients with various skin types. With experience the clinician will be able to select the appropriate treatment to suit an individual patient.

Other topical therapy used to treat PPR includes, erythromycin 2% solution applied twice daily. This may be slightly drying and irritant and is probably not as effective as the other topical treatments listed above but has the advantage that it can be used safely in the pregnant patient (see chapter 8). Tretinoin 0.025% cream or lotion or 0.01% gel applied at night has the theoretical advantage of treating both the actinic damage as well as the rosacea, but is poorly tolerated by rosacea patients with dry sensitive skin and should be avoided in pregnancy. Isotretinoin 0.05% and erythromycin 2% alcohol gel applied as a thin film twice daily may also be effective, but again irritancy may reduce its acceptability to patients and it does not appear to have any advantage over the better tolerated metronidazole and azelaic acid products. Other topical therapies that have been reported to be effective in treating individual or small groups of patients with PPR include various sulfur-containing products (often in combination with salicylic acid or precipitated sulfur with 0.75% hydrocortisone lotion), benzoyl peroxide gel (which is quite drying and poorly tolerated on the rosacea patient's skin) sometimes used in combination with clindamycin 1% or erythromycin, and topical antimite preparations (Permethrin 1% or ivermectin 1.87% creams). There is insufficient evidence to recommend these medications and the clinician is best advised to adhere to the FDA approved and appropriately tested products. Only in the exceptional case will it be necessary to resort to any of these latter agents. Topical calcineurin antagonists such as tacrolimus and pimecrolimus initially showed promise in the treatment of PPR, but they may induce a rosaceiform eruption (as already discussed) and so their use for these patients should probably be avoided. The method of application of topical therapies and how they should be used in relation to cosmetic and sun-block creams is covered in chapter 8.

When the eruption is florid with intense erythema and multiple papules and pustules, or if plaques are present (graded as severe), it is probably wisest to commence treatment with a systemic antibiotic medication as the inflamed skin may be poorly tolerant of surface therapies. The choice of antibiotic to prescribe, the optimum dosage and the required duration of therapy has not been well established and a variety of medications have been suggested (Table 3). Long clinical experience

Table 3 Systemic Treatments for PPR

Permethrina (cream) Systemic medications: Oxytetracycline
Doxycycline
Minocycline
Erythromycin
Clarithromycin
Metronidazole[a]
Trimethoprim[a]
Isotretinoin[a]
Zinc sulfate[a]
Azithomycin[a]
Ivermectin[a] (cream or systemically)
Permethrin[a] (cream)
Photodynamic therapy[a]
Laser therapy (useful for persistent telangiectasias)

[a]The validity of these treatments is unproven.

supports the effectiveness of tetracycline (or related medications). Oxytetracycline (in a dosage of 500 mgs twice daily over 6 to 8 weeks) was one of the first antibiotics used to treat PPR and is effective (and cheap!) for many patients. Problems with absorption, gastrointestinal tolerance and candidiasis limit patient's tolerance of this drug. Doxycycline 100 mgs twice daily for the same duration appears to be equally effective. Patients taking these medications should be cautioned regarding possible photosensitive reactions. A promising recent development has been the approval of low dosage ("sub-antimicrobial") doxycycline which may reduce the propensity to develop vaginal candidiasis that is a distressing side effect of antibiotic therapy in some women. Minocycline is usually well tolerated by patients and appears to act more rapidly than other antibiotics (possibly related to its lipophilic properties and penetration of the pilosebaceous follicle), but it is expensive and can rarely lead to unsightly hyper pigmentation of the skin (which can persist after discontinuing treatment) or headaches (benign intracranial hypertension) and should not be used for prolonged periods without appropriate monitoring. Erythromycin 500 mgs twice daily) is a useful alternative and can be used (if systemic treatment is considered essential) in the pregnant patient. The above mentioned should probably be considered as the "front-line" systemic treatments of PPR. The duration of systemic treatment required to control the inflammatory papules and pustules of PPR ranges from 6 to 12 weeks. Some patients will notice a more rapid response with the skin settling within three weeks, while occasionally a patient will fail to respond to one of the systemic agents shown in Table 2 and may need to be changed to another. There is rarely a complete lack of response to systemic antibiotic therapy, although sometimes patients report that an antibiotic that formerly was effective in controlling their eruption has become ineffective, as if they have developed "resistance" to that treatment. As with topical therapy the choice of which systemic therapy to prescribe often depends on the physician's previous experience and on the particular patient that is being treated. Thus, some systemic treatments are contraindicated in pregnant or lactating women and may reduce the effectiveness of oral contraceptives, others may be excluded because of gastrointestinal intolerance or because the patient is taking concurrent medications that could interact with the rosacea therapy, and sometimes the cost of the medication is a factor.

Second line treatments include macrolides such as clarithromycin and azithromycin which may have a more rapid action and less tendency to gastrointestinal side effects than erythromycin. Trimethoprim 200 mg twice daily for six weeks appears to give excellent results, but the evidence to support its use is lacking and it is more likely to cause allergic skin eruptions than the other oral medications discussed here. It must be avoided in pregnancy, as it is a folate antagonist. In patients who fail to respond to first or second line systemic treatments consideration should be given to the use of other agents. Metronidazole 200 mg twice daily is effective for severe PPR but neurologic side effects and its drug-interaction profile limit its use to exceptional cases only.

Occasionally a patient whose PPR is resistant to systemic antibiotic therapy will respond to treatment with isotretinoin. Caution is needed in the use of this drug for the management of PPR because (in addition to its other potentially serious side effects) the drying effects of isotretinoin on the skin and conjunctiva are poorly tolerated by these patients and a low-dosage regimen is needed (see chap. 1). In addition (unlike the response in acne vulgaris) the improvement gained by patients with PPR following isotretinoin treatment is usually short lived. The other treatments shown in Table 3 are based on reports of individual or small series of patient responses and are provided for information only. As with topical therapy, the physician is advised to familiarize themselves with the side-effect profiles of two or three systemic therapies of rosacea and then select the appropriate treatment based on the requirements of the individual patient under their care. A complete lack of response to more than one systemic agent should prompt a review of the diagnosis. Skin scrapings, skin biopsy, skin surface biopsy, patch test, photopatch tests, etc., may then be considered as appropriate (Table 1).

Once the acute inflammation has subsided in a patient with severe PPR, treatment with a topical agent should be added before discontinuing systemic therapy and used for at least 4 months as "maintenance treatment" after systemic treatment is stopped. In some patients reintroduction of systemic therapy will be required from time to time to maintain remission, while others will be able to keep their skin under good control with topical therapy only.

If the patient remains clear after 4 months the frequency of application can be reduced and (if no flare occurs) topical medication discontinued. However, there is often relapse of the papules and pustules (this occurs within three months of discontinuing topical treatment in the majority of cases) and topical (and/or systemic) treatment then needs to be reintroduced. There is an argument for continuing topical therapy indefinitely in order to avoid the occurrence of such flares. However, the only way to evaluate disease activity levels and avoid unnecessary medication usage is to discontinue treatment temporarily and reintroduce if required.

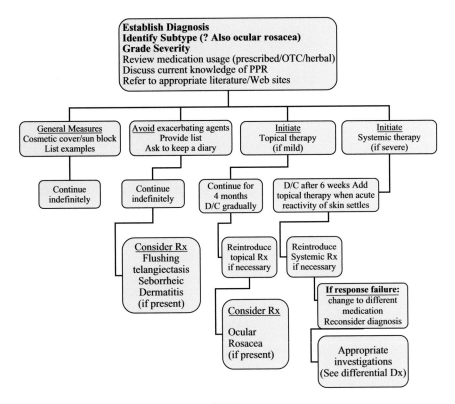

Algorithm 1   Algorithm management of PPR

Other therapeutic approaches that may be necessary in individual patients with PPR include laser therapy for telangiectasias, oxymetazoline for persistent erythema, cosmetic camouflage and counselling for psychologically affected individuals. Recently, the use of photodynamic therapy for patients with PPR has been reported (15). The future role of this treatment in the management of patients with PPR remains to be determined, but it offers a potential option in those individuals who are unable to tolerate other forms of treatment.

The overall approach to the management of a patient with PPR is summarized in the algorithm 1.

KEY POINTS

- PPR is usually easily diagnosed on the clinical appearance of erythema, papules and pustules in a centrofacial distribution.
- If the distribution is atypical consider alternative diagnoses.
- Mild to moderate PPR responds well to topical medications.
- First line topical treatments are metronidazole and azelaic acid preparations
- Topical erythromycin is helpful for the patient who is pregnant.
- Topical treatment should be continued for a minimum of 4 months.

- Relapse often occurs when topical therapy is stopped.
- Tetracycline and related antibiotics are well established systemic treatments for PPR.
- Systemic therapy should be continued for a minimum of 4 weeks.
- Patients may have to be changed from one topical or systemic treatment to another if the response is inadequate.

REFERENCES

1. Kligman AM. Ocular rosacea. Arch Dermatol 1997; 133:89–90.
2. Sneddon I. Perioral dermatitis. Brit J Dermatol 1973; 87:430–434.
3. Marks R, Wilson Jones E. Disseminated rosacea. Br J Dermatol 1969; 81:16–27.
4. Wilson Erasmus. Diseases of the Skin. London, 1842.
5. Plumbe S. Diseases of the Skin, 4th ed. London, 1837.
6. Brinnel H, Friedel J, Caputa M, et al. Rosacea: Disturbed defense against brain overheating. Arch Dermatol Res 1989; 281:66–72.
7. Jones MP, Knable AL, White MJ, et al. Helicobacter pylori in rosacea: Lack of an association. Arch Dermatol 1998; 134:511.
8. Lacey N, Delaney S, Kavanagh K, et al. Mite-related bacterial antigens stimulate inflammatory cells in rosacea. Brit J Dermatol 2007; 157:474–481.
9. Antille C, Saurat JH, Lubbe J. Induction of rosaceiform dermatitis during treatment of facial inflammatory dermatoses with tacrolimus ointment. Arch Dermatol 2004; 140:457–460.
10. Bonner E, Eustace P, Powell FC. The demodex mite population in rosacea. J Am Acad Dermatol 1993; 28: 443–448.
11. Poulos GA, Brodell RT. Perioral dermatitis associated with an inhaled corticosteroid. Arch Dermatol 2007; 143:1460.
12. Forton F, Germaux MA, Brasseur T, et al. Demodicosis and rosacea: Epidemiology and significance in daily dermatologic practice. J Am Acad Dermatol 2005; 52:74–87.
13. McAleer M, Powell FC. Complementary and alternative medicine usage in rosacea. Btir J Dermatol 2008; 158:1134–1173.
14. Powell FC. Rosacea. N Eng J Med 2005; 352: 793–803.
15. Nybaek H, Jemec GBE. Photodynamic therapy in the treatment of rosacea. Dermatology 2005; 211:135–138.

FURTHER READING

J Drugs Dermatol 2006; 5(Issue 1).

Comment: This journal contains excellent review articles on topical therapy for rosacea (by Nally and Berson) and oral treatments (by Baldwin). Consult these for in-depth review of these subjects.

Wakelin SH. Handbook of systemic drug treatment in Dermatology. Manson Publishing. 2002.

Comment: This is a handy, compact reference source dealing only with drugs used to treat dermatology patients. The section on acne deals with many of the treatments used for rosacea patients.

6

Phymatous (Subtype 3) Rosacea

"When God was giving out noses,
I thought he said "roses"!
And asked for a big red one!"
  Said to his grandson by a patient to explain his rhinophyma

"Le viola donc, ce nez, qui des traits de son maître
A détruit l'harmonie! Il en rougit, le traître!"
                    E. Rostand, *Cyrano de Bergerac*

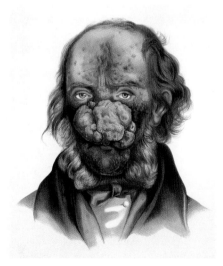

Figure 1   Early illustration of rhinophyma showing gross nasal deformity in a middle-aged man. The nasal distortion in this patient is such that one has to wonder if there has been the development of a carcinoma in the nasal tissue. Note also the erythematous papules and pustules of PPR on his forehead and the erythema of the medial cheeks.

DEFINITION

Phymatous rosacea is a persistent, firm, non-painful, non-pitting swelling of the tissue of the nose (rhinophyma), chin (gnathophyma), ears (otophyma), forehead (mentophyma), or eyelids (blepharophyma). The clinical picture of persistent edema and phymatous changes may overlap in some patients. Swelling is often associated with erythema and sometimes with other manifestations of rosacea (papules, pustules, and telangiectasias), and occasionally ocular inflammation.

DISTRIBUTION

The distribution of the phymatous involvement depends on the area involved, as outlined above. Rhinophyma is often apparent initially at the distal end of the nose as dilated patulous follicles. When rhinophyma becomes marked, it leads to the greatest deformity in this region. Gnathophyma is a rare occurrence with the central chin typically being involved, while the lower half of the helices of the ears and the lobes are mainly affected in otophyma. Edema in this region may be present in severe inflammatory papulopustular rosacea (Fig. 2) but is often overlooked. The forehead is centrally involved in mentophyma (described as being a cushion-like swelling and seen in side view in fig 10) that can also sometimes be seen in patients with facial edema and rosacea when the swelling extends to the medial cheeks and the periocular region. Blepharophyma refers to the swelling of the eyelids, which is usually seen as a component of edematous rosacea, or which may accompany severe papulopustular or ocular rosacea (Fig. 3).

Practice Point: The edema of this man's face (Fig. 3) was so severe that when he awoke in the morning he had to spend several minutes massaging the swelling away from his eyes in order to see properly. He found this as the only effective method reducing his facial swelling. He had in addition moderate PPR which responded well to topical and systemic antibitic therapy, but the edema and swelling persisted unchanged apart from minor fluctuations.

   Comment: Some individuals, usually men, seem to be prone to developing edema with inflammatory rosacea. Although this patient was unaware of it, facial massage therapy for rosacea had been proposed by the great Scandanavian dermatologist Sobye in a publication over fifty years earlier. Is this another treatment method that needs reevaluation?

BACKGROUND

Because phymatous rosacea apart from rhinophyma is so rarely encountered by practitioners, the following discussion will be limited to the latter condition. First described by Hebra in 1845, rhinophyma is one of the most easily recognized subtypes of rosacea. Rhinophyma is sometimes considered to be the end point or most advanced type of rosacea, but it can occur in patients who otherwise have mild rosacea or even in those without any other evidence of the disease

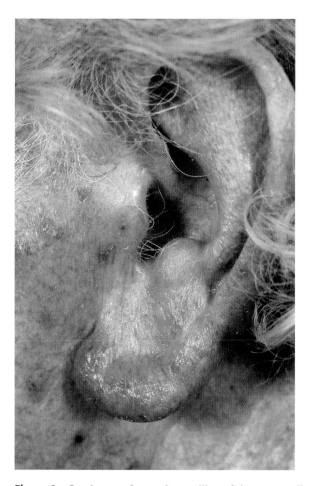

Figure 2 Otophyma refers to the swelling of the ear, usually most marked on the lobe. It is seen here in a patient with severe PPR some lesion of which are visible on the lateral cheek.

whatsoever. There is no consistent relationship between the duration, severity, or any other feature of rosacea and the occurrence of rhinophyma. There may be a genetic propensity toward the development of rhinophyma, as sometimes more than one family member may be affected. Rhinophyma should therefore more accurately be designated as a condition of the skin that is closely associated with rosacea rather than a disorder that occurs as a consequence of the disease. There are several different forms of rhinophyma as listed in Table 1 (1).

Rhinophyma is fortunately a rare malady. Sadly the deformity seems to inspire amusement and a sense of ridicule in some observers, rather than sympathy and understanding that the sufferer deserves. This is compounded by the fallacious association in the mind of some of the general public and the physicians of the past between rhinophyma and the abuse of alcohol. Thus, titles such as "whiskey nose,"

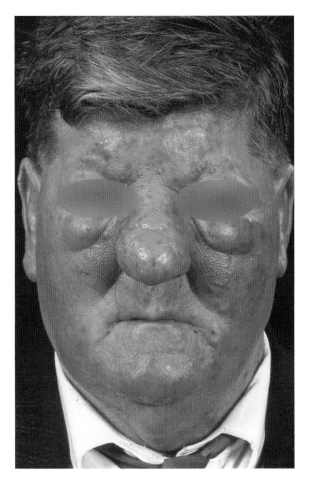

Figure 3   Blepharophyma is the term applied to persistent swelling of the eyelids and periorbital tissue. It is most evident in this patient as an infra- orbital swelling. Note also the prominent glandular rhinophyma with nodular deformities.

"brandy nose," "rum blossom," "le nez des Buveurs," have been used as labels for rhinophyma in the older medical literature. The location of rhinophyma on the most prominent part of the face has maximized the negative cosmetic impact of this disorder and increased the social stigmatization of patients with rhinophyma. Another aspect of rhinophyma that places it in a different category from the other rosacea subtypes is the occasional occurrence of malignant change in the affected nasal skin. Although rarely reported, both basal and squamous cell carcinomas can occur in affected skin of patients with rhinophyma, so the clinician should have a low threshold for taking a biopsy of new or unstable outgrowths of the nose in these patients.

Table 1 Forms of Rhinophyma

Form	Description
Glandular	Commonest and most disfiguring. Increased prominence of follicular orifices and sebum secretion in mild cases. Often asymmetrical nodular outgrowths of tissue in severe forms.
Angiomatous	Usually in fair-skinned patients. Dark red to purple color of the nose may adopt an acrocyanotic hue in cold weather. Splayed vessels initially seen on alae nasi extend to dorsum of nose in advanced cases.
Actinic	A yellowish discoloration, sebaceous hyperplasia, an irregular surface of the skin, and actinic comedones are features. Rarely enlarges major degree.
Acneform	Occurs in older (usually male) patients with longstanding acne vulgaris. Oily skin, comedones, cysts, and scarring are features of the surrounding skin.
Fibrous	Diffuse hyperplasia of connective tissue gives a firm texture to the enlarged nose.
Obstructive	Not a true rhinophyma. Occurs in individuals who wear spectacles that cause deep indentations and possibly lymphatic obstruction. Mucin may be detected histologically.

CLINICAL FEATURES

One of the most striking clinical features of rhinophyma is its predilection for male patients. In contrast to the other rosacea variants, which are found with equal frequency in both males and females, rhinophyma occurs almost 20 times more commonly in male patients. The reason for this is unknown, but male patients with rosacea may be more likely to have oily skin and evidence of sebaceous hyperplasia.

The first clinical signs of the commonest type of rhinophyma (called the **glandular** form) are usually seen in the skin of the alae nasi and distal dorsal nose. The follicular openings in these areas appear enlarged and become more prominent (sometimes referred to as being "patulous") even before there is a detectable increase in the size of the nose. The dark color of the oxygenated sebum at the follicular orifices further highlights these pores. The next change is a mild but definite bulbous swelling of the nose with a "peau d'orange" appearance of the skin developing as the pores that are seen as indentations due to the surrounding tissue distention (Fig. 4). More distinctive swelling of the nose is seen in Figure 5 and again in Figure 6, with increasingly deep indentations between enlarging areas of the distal third of the nose. There is often asymmetry of the nasal swelling, which heightens the abnormal appearance of the nose (Fig. 7). At this stage, the cosmetic impact becomes very significant and the patient is constantly reminded of the changes in the nose by the reactions of those they socially interact with. The ultimate expression of glandular rhinophyma is the development of nodular outgrowths of

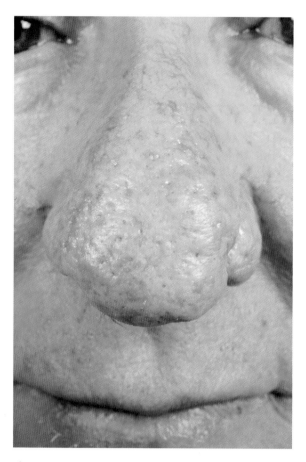

Figure 4 Large follicular openings are prominent on the dorsal surface of this patient's nose with the early swelling of rhinophyma and so called "patulous follicles." These give the skin a "peau d'orange" appearance typical of early glandular rhinophyma.

the nose that distort the appearance of the nose completely (Fig. 8) and which can extend to the nasofacial sulci. Patients with this degree of rhinophyma also frequently complain of an unpleasant odor from the skin, probably arising from the increased sebum production in the tissue overgrowths, and sometimes also from the frequent, mild, secondary bacterial or yeast growth that can occur in the deep fissures between the deforming outgrowths of tissue. Seborrheic dermatitis, which accompanies glandular rhinophyma in some patients, may contribute to the yeast population on the skin as well as the cosmetic impact because of the accompanying scale and erythema.

As mentioned earlier, the possibility of basal or squamous cell carcinoma developing in rhinophyma has to be borne in mind, and any rapidly progressive lesion, or lesions that become eroded or ulcerated demand that consideration be given to this possibility (Fig. 9).

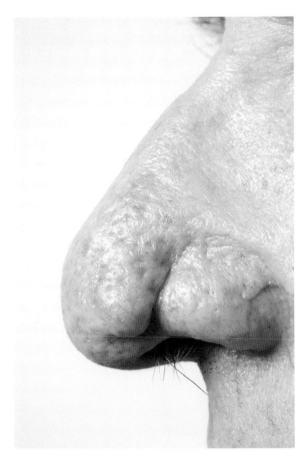

Figure 5   As the nasal enlargement progresses, the swelling becomes more pronounced, sometimes with telangiectatic surface vessels and the development of folds or deep indentations in the enlarging tissue as seen here. The follicular openings remain prominent.

The **angiomatous** form of rhinophyma usually occurs as an isolated finding, but it can be seen in patients who have either subtypes 1 or 2 rosacea. Patients with this form of rhinophyma usually have fair, sun-sensitive types 1 or 2 skin. Small vessels are initially seen at the alae nasi. In time, these vessels enlarge becoming more marked and contributing to the redness of the nose (see Fig. 7 in chapter 4). Sometimes the nose in angiomatous rhinophyma has a distinctive cyanotic hue. The nasal swelling of angiomatous rhinophyma is less than that seen in patients with glandular rhinophyma, and distortion is not usually a feature.

Some patients who have types 2 or 3 skin react to chronic climatic exposure and weathering by developing thickened "leathery" skin which has a yellowish discolored appearance. Such patients may develop nasal swelling to a degree that they are classified as having the **actinic** form of rhinophyma. The yellowish nasal

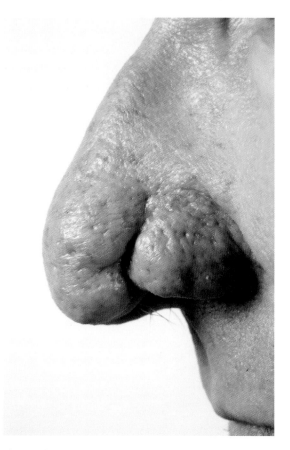

Figure 6 This patient shows similar but more progressive signs of rhinophyma compared to the changes illustrated in Fig. 5 with deep furrowing and tissue distension and the beginning of nodular deformity. Note the prominent dilated "patulous" follicles.

swelling often has an irregular surface due to areas of sebaceous hyperplasia and large actinic comedones are prominent (sometimes called "potato nose"). Gross nasal distortion rarely occurs (Fig. 10).

Occasionally, older patients with persistent **acne** vulgaris develop a form of rhinophyma. Oily skin, comedones, cysts, and scarring are features that should suggest this diagnosis.

The various forms of rhinophyma together with a synopsis of their clinical features are shown in Table 1.

HISTOPATHOLOGY

The histopathologic changes seen in skin biopsies from patients with glandular rhinophyma are distinctive (2). The epidermis usually appears normal with the exception of large follicular openings some of which may appear to be plugged

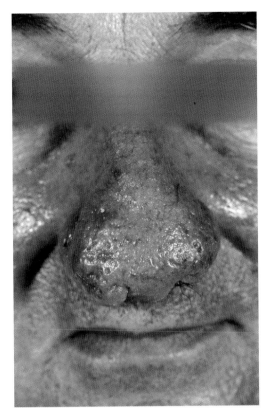

Figure 7 The asymmetry of the nasal swelling is well shown in this view of another patient with evolving rhinophyma, mainly involving the right side of his nose. Some patients with glandular rhinophyma squeeze the oily secretions from the pores of their nose, which they often refer to as looking like "small white worms" coming out of their skin. It is important to reassure them that this is semi-solid sebum.

by sebaceous material. An undulating appearance of the epidermis may be seen in patients with nodular outgrowths of the nose. The follicular openings often appear widely dilated and the canals distended with sebum and may contain numerous demodex mites. Inflammatory changes are mild or absent unless there is secondary infection or concomitant inflammatory papules or pustules of PPR. Telangiectatic vessels may be seen, being marked in patients with the vascular form of rhinophyma. Granulomatous changes are only seen if there is advanced follicular inflammation with rupture. The most striking findings are seen in the mid and deep dermis. In these areas there are multiple aggregates of sebaceous gland hyperplasia in an asymmetrical distribution the morphology of which otherwise appear normal. The proliferation of these glands causes the swelling and distortion of the nose. A similar histological appearance is seen in patients with sebaceous adenomas or isolated areas of sebaceous hyperplasia, so clinicopathological

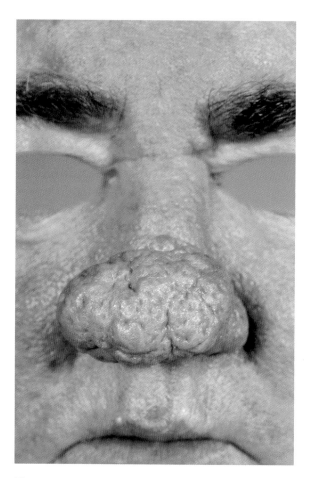

Figure 8 Gross distortion of nose is seen in this man with advanced rhinophyma. He only ever had mild accompanying PPR, contradicting the assertion that rhinophyma represents the terminal point or "end stage" of severe inflammatory rosacea.

correlation is important in making the diagnosis of glandular rhinophyma. There is often overgrowth of connective tissue with fibrous tracts running through the dermis some of which correspond with the fissures seen clinically between the nodular outgrowths. The histopathological changes in some patients are characterized by marked fibrosis in the superficial and reticular dermis, accentuated around follicles and increased numbers of fibroblasts, while others (especially the obstructive form) show deposition of mucin in the dermis. The collagen in the upper dermis often shows changes of solar elastosis which is marked in patients with rhinophyma secondary to actinic damage.

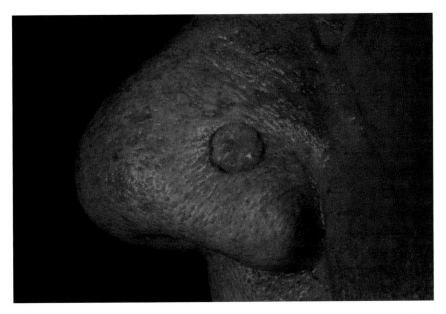

Figure 9 A small basal cell carcinoma is seen here occurring close to the alae nasi on the left side of this patient's nose. He was referred for treatment of mild accompanying rhinophyma. The carcinoma was assumed to be a part of the rhinophyma rather than a separate problem.

Table 2 Differential Diagnosis of Rhinophyma

Condition	Features
Lupus pernio (Sarcoid)	Shiny brown/red/violaceous firm swelling of nose. May be asymmetrical. May extend to medial cheeks. Dioscopy and biopsy help establish diagnosis. Workup for systemic involvement required.
Basal or squamous cell carcinoma	Both may mimic or occur in association with rhinophyma. Rapid growth and surface erosion or ulceration requires biopsy.
Lymphoma/angiosarcoma	Rare. Intranasal biopsy may be necessary to diagnose lymphoma.
Lupus vulgaris (TB)	Now rare in western countries. Can mimic rhinophyma but scarring often present. Biopsy with special studies for diagnosis.
Acrocyanosis	Bluish discoloration of nose, especially in cold weather. Usually no deformity.
Lupus erythematosis	Erythema, scaling, and a tendency to scarring are features of discoid lupus erythematosis.

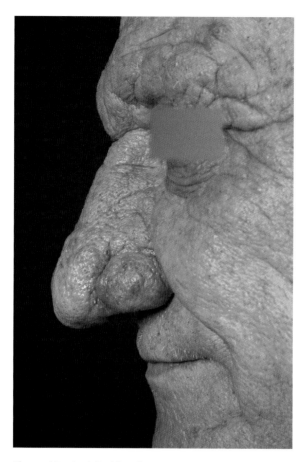

Figure 10   Actinic rhinophyma showing the yellowish discoloration of the enlarged nose together with large actinic comedones and an irregular skin surface due to sebaceous hyperplasia. Note the deep furrowing at both inner and outer angles of the left eye as well as on the medial upper nose, indicating the degree of sebaceous hyperplasia. This patient also shows a degree of mentophyma.

DIFFERENTIAL DIAGNOSIS AND INVESTIGATIONS

The main conditions which should be considered when a patient presents with progressive nasal swelling are shown in Table 2. Lupus pernio (sarcoid of the nose) causes a swelling and distortion of the nose that closely mimics and that may be misdiagnosed as rhinophyma. Careful inspection of the skin in these patients shows a shiny appearance to the skin surface. The large follicular openings containing oxygenated sebum that are the features of rhinophyma are absent. The nose in patients with lupus pernio often has a deep red or a purplish color (Fig. 11), while in patients with glandular rhinophyma, the normal flesh color or a minor degree of erythema of the nose is typically seen. Palpation of the nose reveals a firm, slightly indurated consistency in lupus pernio. In patients with glandular

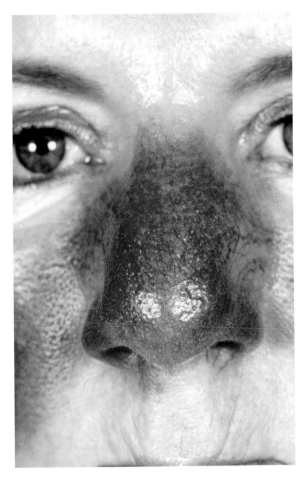

Figure 11 Lupus Pernio (sarcoid of the nose) is characterized by firm, nontender nasal enlargement, which has a dark red to violaceous color. Although follicular openings are preserved to a degree, the patulous follicles of rhinophyma are absent.

rhinophyma the swollen nose feels softer. The use of dioscopy (pressing a glass slide or transparent plastic implement firmly on the affected skin surface) reveals the characteristic "apple jelly nodules" in lupus pernio. These represent the non-caseating dermal granulomas that are the histologic hallmark of this disorder. The diagnosis of sarcoid should be confirmed by a skin biopsy, which typically shows the dermal granulomas with little surrounding inflammation (sometimes called "naked granulomas"). Other appropriate investigations (chest X-ray, pulmonary function studies, ocular examination, etc.) should be carried out if the diagnosis is confirmed to determine if there is multisystem involvement and referral to an appropriate specialist as required.

One of the most important considerations in a patient with rhinophyma is to exclude the possibility of malignancy. As indicated earlier, patients with glandular rhinophyma seem to have a predisposition to the development of basal and squamous cell carcinomas of the nose. Thus, one or even several biopsies of any new, rapidly changing, or suspicious growths should be taken. Nasal lymphomas have also been mistaken for rhinophyma, and in these cases intranasal mucosal biopsies may need to be taken to establish the diagnosis with certainty (3) (Fig. 12). Consultation with an Otolaryngologist may be necessary if this diagnosis is a

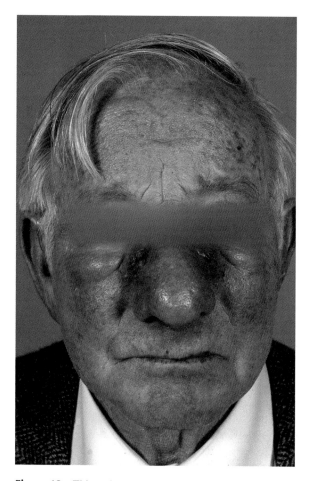

Figure 12 This patient had a nasal lymphoma that was initially mistaken for rhinophyma. Note the swelling of the cheeks and the marked infra-orbital swellings which developed in conjunction with the progressive nasal enlargement. Several cutaneous and intranasal biopsies were required to establish the diagnosis of large cell lymphoma of the nose. This subsequently cleared with chemotherapy (3).

consideration. Sebaceous carcinoma and angiosarcoma are other rare neoplasms that have been mistaken for rhinophyma.

> **Practice Point:** This man (Fig. 12) was referred for treatment of rhinophyma. He gave a history of a progressive enlargement of his nose over the previous 18 months. This was associated with considerable discomfort. Examination revealed firm, shiny induration of the distal nasal tissue with swelling of the upper face.
>
> *Comment: The atypical history combined with the unusual clinical features suggested further investigation. Several cutaneous and intranasal biopsies were required to confirm the diagnosis of lymphoma. If the history, or clinical features, do not fit, or if there is a or lack of response to treatment think again and institute appropriate investigations.*

Other conditions that have been confused with rhinophyma are shown in Table 2. The possibility of infection, including deep fungal and mycobacterial infection, (Fig. 13) as well as abnormal presentations of autoimmune disease, such as discoid lupus erythematosus, (Fig. 14) must be considered in some patients.

MANAGEMENT

Isotretinoin has been used as a medical treatment for the early clinical signs of glandular rhinophyma (4). It may be best suited for those patients who have inflammatory changes (papules and pustules) and oily greasy skin (seborrhea) as well as rhinophyma. There have been conflicting reports as to the efficacy of this treatment (which may be used in combination with dermabrasion). Because only small numbers of patients have been treated with this agent, the optimum dosage to prescribe, the duration of therapy, and the long-term outcome is unclear. Dapsone is another medication which has been used to treat rhinophyma. It probably exercises its effect on accompanying inflammatory lesions with associated edematous changes and there is insufficient supportive evidence to recommend its use.

Pulsed dye laser obliteration of the prominent vessels in the angiomatous form of rhinophyma can be very effective. The nasal erythema markedly diminishes and scarring rarely occurs. The CO_2 laser is also an effective treatment modality for rhinophyma, those with the glandular form benefiting most. Even large distorting nodules can be successfully destroyed with this laser and the cosmetic appearance of the end results is surprisingly good (5). A variety of traditional "cold steel" surgical approaches are also effective in the treatment of the nodules of advanced glandular rhinophyma. These include simple shave excision and razor modeling with subsequent healing by granulation and reepithelization,

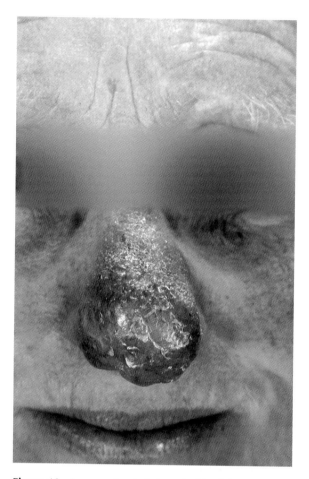

Figure 13 Lupus vulgaris (tuberculosis) of the distal nose is shown in this patient. The unusual color and firm consistency of the nose, scarring and the absence of patulous follicles and the prominent surface scale are against the diagnosis of rhinophyma. Dioscopy indicated the presence of granulomas. Histologic and subsequent microbiologic evaluation established the diagnosis.

subepidermal debridement and debulking with electrosurgery, as well as excision and direct suture or excision and grafting (usually with skin taken from the supraclavicular region). It is important that most but not all sebaceous hyperplasia be removed, as overzealous removal of sebaceous tissue seems to heighten the risk of postoperative scarring. Other treatments that have been reported in individual patients or small series of patients with rhinophyma include electrodessication, dermabrasion, cryosurgery, and radiation therapy.

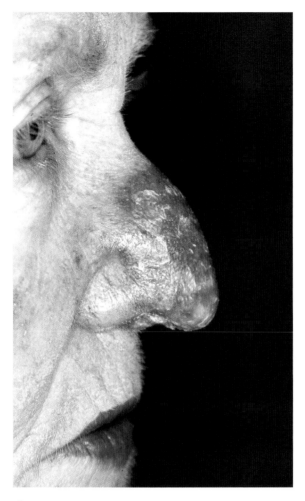

Figure 14 The prominent surface scale, the shiny scarred appearance of the skin surface, and the lack of patulous follicles were all clinical indications of the presence of discoid lupus erythematosus in this middle-aged female patient. Skin biopsies for histology and direct immunofluoresence were required to establish the diagnosis.

KEY POINTS

- A range of phymatous changes may be seen is patients with rosacea.
- Rhinophyma is the commonest phymatous change and is the most susceptible to treatment.
- Rhinophyma occurs mainly in male patients and there are several clinical varients

- Rhinophyma does not represent the "end point" of progressive inflammation in rosacea patients and may occur with little (or even no) preceding inflammation
- Other conditions must be considered in the differential diagnosis of progressive nasal enlargement and appropriate investigations undertaken
- Laser and surgical approaches are effective treatments for rhinophyma

REFERENCES

1. Jansen T, Plewig G. Miscellaneous rosacea disorders. In: Demis DJ, ed. Clinical Dermatology, Vol. 2. Lippincott-Raven, 1997: section 10–8, pp. 1–7.
2. Aloi F, Tomasini C, Soro E, et al. The Clinicopathologic spectrum of rhinophyma. J Am Acad Dermatol 2000; 42:468–472.
3. Murphy A, O'Keane JC, Blayney A, et al. Cutaneous presentation of nasal lymphoma: A report of two cases. J Am Acad Dermatol 1998; 38:310–313.
4. Rodder O, Plewig G. Rhinophyma and rosacea: Combined treatment with isotretinoin and dermabrasion. In: Acne and Rosacea: Proceedings of a Symposium 1988 Martin Dunitz 1988:335–338.
5. Roenigk R. CO_2 Laser vaporization for treatment of Rhinophyma. Mayo Clinic Proc 1987; 62:676–680.

FURTHER READING

Rolleston JD. A note on the early history of rhinophyma. Proc R Soc Med 1932; 26: 327–329.

Comment: This an interesting read about the early descriptions of rosacea.

Sobye P. Treatment of rosacea by massage. Acta Derm Venereol 1951; 31:174–183.

Comment: A well-written article by this recognized authority on rosacea. Such treatments may have their place in the management of some patients with rosacea and facial swelling (see practice point in this chapter).

7

Ocular Rosacea (Subtype 4)

"The Rabbit-eye of Rosacea"
Gerd Plewig

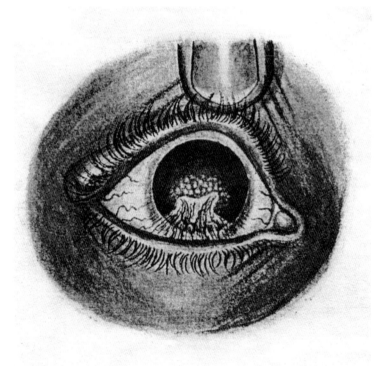

Figure 1   An early illustration of the changes (puntatae ketatopathy, conjunctival injection and conjunctival overgrowth) on to the cornea attributed to severe ocular rosacea.

DEFINITION

Probably the first description of ocular rosacea was by the famous English dermatologist Willan in the early 1800's whose handwritten note on an illustration of a patient with PPR documented the presence of ocular inflammation. Ocular rosacea may be defined as a range of changes that occur in the eye lid, eye lashes or eyes of patients with rosacea. While there are no specific or diagnostic types of ocular inflammation that occur in this condition, some findings and lesions occur commonly. Ocular changes may accompany the skin changes, precede them or follow the appearance of their appearance. Patients with papulopustular rosacea (PPR) appear to be more prone to developing ocular rosacea than those with erythematotelangiectatic rosacea (ETTR) or phymatous rosacea (PR). The duration or severity of ocular rosacea does not appear to parallel the type, duration, or severity of the skin changes, although it has been suggested that there is a correlation between the presence of ocular involvement and the tendency to flush (1). There is no laboratory or investigative test that will confirm the diagnosis of ocular rosacea.

DISTRIBUTION

The structure of the normal eyelid is shown in Figure 2. It is composed of cutaneous, muscular, tarsal, and conjunctival layers. The tarsal layer is made up of

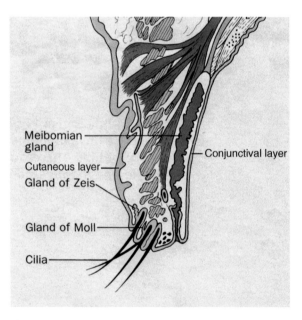

Figure 2 Diagrammatic representation of a cross section of a normal eyelid showing the various structures and their relationships. Note the large meibomian gland and the much smaller glands of Moll and Zeis.

dense fibrous connective tissue that contains the modified sebaceous (meibomian) glands. These glands are commonly dysfunctional in patients with rosacea. The ocular disorders seen in patients with rosacea may affect any of the following sections of the eye or related structures:

- The margins of the eyelids (blepharitis/conical dandruff/telangiectasias of lid margins).
- The conjunctiva (conjunctivitis/conjunctival injection/conjunctival overgrowth).
- The glands of Zeiss (hordeolum externum).
- The meibomian glands (reduced tear breakup time/thickened secretions/plugged "capped" orifices/chalazion/hordeolum internum/).
- The lacrimal glands (reduced aqueous tear secretion).
- The cornea (punctuate epithelial erosions/keratitis/perforation).
- Sclera (scleritis/episcleritis) the uvea (uveitis).
- Iris (iritis).

Mild disorders are common, while serious ocular disease is rare in patients with rosacea.

BACKGROUND

Rosacea is almost unique among the inflammatory dermatoses in that it is often accompanied by ocular inflammation or dysfunction. The reason for this is unknown. The ocular changes seen in patients with rosacea are not distinctive to rosacea and the diagnosis of ocular rosacea cannot be made with certainty in the absence of cutaneous changes. As the ocular disorders may precede the onset of those in the skin, this means that in these patients the definitive diagnosis can only be made retrospectively. The frequency with which ocular changes in patients with rosacea is reported in the literature ranges from 20% to 60%, depending on whether the findings are being recorded by dermatologists or ophthalmologists.

The commonest ocular involvement in patients with rosacea is probably dysfunction of the meibomian glands. Meibomian glands lie within the tarsal plates of the upper and lower lids (Fig. 2). Their openings (approximately 30 on each lid margin) are visible behind the eyelashes (cilia). Meibomian glands are considered to be modified sebaceous glands and are responsible for the production of the outer lipid layer of the tear film. Their oily secretions (made up largely of waxes and sterol esters) spread over the lid margins. Alteration in the composition of these secretions may result in ocular changes. An increase in the proportion of free fatty acids in the tear film can cause conjunctival hyperaemia and punctate corneal epithelial breakdown. The tear film has an important role in maintaining the health of the ocular surface through lubrication, lavage, supply of nutrients, removal of debris, and probably by antimicrobial activity. It is a dynamic three layered substance composed of an outer lipid layer, a middle aqueous layer (derived from the lacrimal glands) and an inner mucous layer secreted by conjunctival goblet cells. The tear film is unstable and the meibomian gland derived outer lipid layer is an important element as it helps to maintain the integrity of the tear film and prevent its rapid evaporation. The time it takes for the tear film to degenerate (called the "tear breakup time") has implications for the integrity of the surface ocular environment. It is defined as the amount of time it takes for a random dry spot to appear in the tear film after a blink and is visualized using a flourescine dye. A normal tear breakup time is considered to be greater than 10 seconds and can be reduced in hot, dry or windy conditions. Studies of patients with ocular rosacea have consistently shown that the tear breakup time is reduced to approximately 50% of normal, and the severity of ocular symptoms is inversely proportional to the breakup time, i.e., the lower the tear breakup time the more severe the symptoms (2). The reduced tear breakup time may be normalized after systemic treatment of rosacea using doxycycline. In some patients with rosacea, the openings of the meibomian glands appear plugged or "capped" with inspissated secretions. The obstruction of these openings have at times to be removed physically to allow the secretions to flow freely. The viscous secretions in patients with rosacea may facilitate the multiplication of demodex mites which frequently infest the lashes of patients with ocular rosacea. Meibomian cysts sometimes occur due to obstruction of meibomian secretions which causes resultant inflammatory changes and a cystic swelling (chalazion) as shown in Figure 3. The aqueous tear production

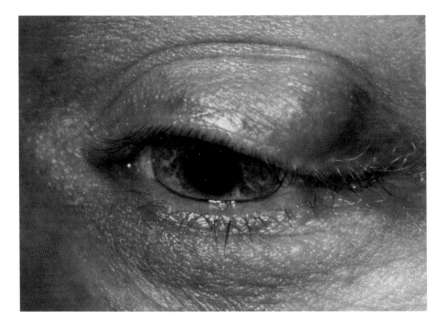

Figure 3   Meibomian gland obstruction is manifested as a prominent swelling of the surface of the upper lid, a typical presentation of a chalazion.

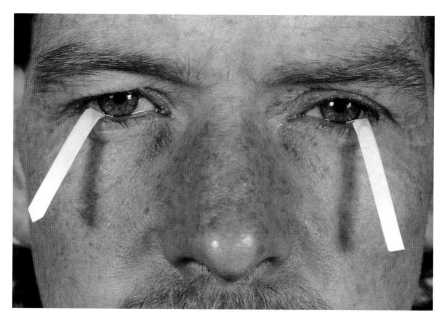

Figure 4 Schirmer testing in a patient who had cutaneous lesions of PPR (cleared with topical metronidazole gel applied twice daily) who also complained of itchy eyes and intermittent inflammation of the left upper lid. The results revealed reduced tear production in both eyes and tear supplementation was prescribed. Tear production may be reduced asymmetrically (more in one eye than another) so it is important to evaluate both.

as measured by the Schirmer test is also reduced in patients with rosacea consistent with patient's frequent complaints of dry eyes (3). Figure 4 demonstrates the use of the Schirmer test in a patient with rosacea. Inflammatory cytokines have been shown to be elevated in the tears of patients with rosacea (4).

Although rarely serious or sight threatening, the symptoms of ocular rosacea are at least irritating and inconvenient for the patient and sometimes quite troublesome. The physician dealing with patients with rosacea should be aware of the varied clinical presentations of ocular involvement and the approach to their management.

"Always look the patient in the eye!

CLINICAL FEATURES

The disparate ocular changes that have been described under the title of "ocular rosacea" are listed in Table 1. One or both eyes may be affected at any given time. Ocular rosacea may affect the (*i*) eyelid margins, (*ii*) the ocular secretions, and (*iii*) the conjunctiva (all common and usually mild) as well as (*iv*) the cornea, (*v*)

Table 1   Clinical Features of Ocular Rosacea

Ocular structure	Presentation
Eyelashes (cilia)	Concretions at the base of the cilia.
	Conical dandruff.
	Loss of lashes.
	Demodex folliculorum visible on lash pluck.
Eyelids	Scaling and crusting of the lid margins (scurf).
	Erythema and swelling of lids in chronic disease.
	Telangiectasias may be visible on lid margins.
Conjunctiva	Conjunctival injection.
	Hyperemic bacterial/viral conjunctivitis.
	May be contagious.
	"Lacey" vessels on tarsal or bulbar conjunctiva.
Meibomian glands	Often dysfunctional.
	Orifices may be capped or plugged.
	Secretions may become thickened and "wormlike". when expressed from the glands.
	Glandular dropout may occur.
	Chalazion presents as painless cystic swelling that distorts eyelid.
	If suppurates becomes painful (hordeolum internum).
Glands of Zeis	Hordeolum externum (stye) presents as swelling with pustulation pointing at a cilia on the lid margin.
Cornea	Mild punctate erosive epithelial keratitis.
	Neovascularisation rare.
	Ulceration or rupture very rare.
Sclera	Scleritis and episcleritis are rare.
	Pain is usually prominent.
Uvea	Uveitis rare.
	Painful and sight threatening.
Iris	As for uvea.

the sclera, or (*vi*) the uvea (all rare and potentially sight threatening). While any of the above areas may be affected in isolation, more than one aspect of ocular function may be affected simultaneously in some patients with ocular rosacea.

Most patients do not volunteer any specific complaint related to their eyes when presenting with the skin changes of rosacea. This is because they are usually mild and they do not relate their eye symptoms to their skin condition. It therefore behooves the clinician to specifically enquire about ocular symptoms. Sometimes, patients with cutaneous lesions of rosacea give a history of having recurrent "cysts" (probably chalazia or hordeola) removed surgically from their eyelids in the past. At other times patients may deny having ocular symptoms, but will relate that they have used liquid tears on a regular basis to relieve symptoms that probably were due to ocular rosacea.

One of the commonest symptoms of ocular rosacea is a mild sensation of itch, burning, stinging, or grittiness in their eyes. These symptoms probably relate to dryness of the eyes and often are worse in winter months and with exposure to cold winds. Often patients dismiss these symptoms as being minor, feel they may have a foreign body in their eyes.

Practice Point: A 42-year-old woman was referred for the treatment of PPR. She denied any ocular symptoms but on direct questioning, she agreed that she had found it "troublesome" to wear her contact lenses (they had irritated her eyes recently) and that she was now inclined to use tear supplements that she did not require previously.

Comment: Symptoms as described by this patient are often not regarded as relevant by patients. Direct questioning is necessary to elicit this information. Low dose doxycycline taken over 6 weeks which was prescribed primarily for PPR restored this woman's ability to wear contact lenses without discomfort and cleared her skin lesions.

Inspection of the eyelid margins rosacea often reveals a slight crusting or scaling indicating the presence of blepharitis (Fig. 13 of chap. 5). In chronic cases, there may be lid swelling and redness (Fig. 5). These changes are not specific for

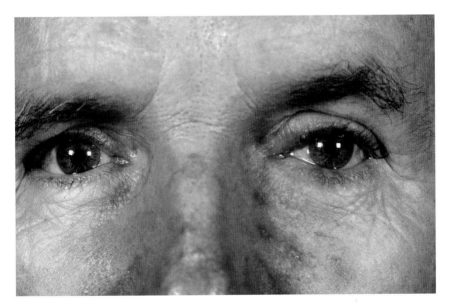

Figure 5 Ocular rosacea is manifested in this middle aged male patient (who also has mild PPR) by the presence of redness and swelling (of the left lower lid mainly) and a chalazion of the left upper lid.

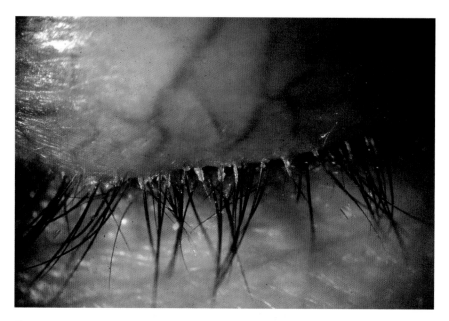

Figure 6 Collarettes of keratin (conical dandruff) are visible at the bases of several of the eye lashes of this patient's upper lid who had mild PPR and complained of irritated eyes.

rosacea and similar crusting can be seen in patients with seborrhoeic dermatitis (which can accompany rosacea in some individuals). In severe cases, there may be loss of lashes. A swab taken from the lid margin in such patients often shows the presence of staphylococcal bacterial overgrowth.

Sometimes a conical sheath of keratin can be seen enveloping the shafts of the cilia (eyelashes) as a kind of collaret around the base of the hairs, so called "conical dandruff" (Fig. 6). These changes are more characteristic of rosacea, and microscopy can sometimes reveal demodex mites encased in the keratin surrounding the lashes at the eyelid margins (Fig. 7). Blocked or inspissated meibomian gland openings may be seen on the tarsal margins, expression of which reveals a "wormlike" viscous material. Individuals with these kinds of changes often complain of a sensation of dryness of their eyes, or paradoxically that their eyes tend to "water" easily when exposed to minor irritants such as cold winds, etc. The "watering" sensation that some of these patients experience may reflect the altered lipid component of the tear film which results in more rapid than normal dissipation of the film.

Dilatation (injection) of the blood vessels of the conjunctiva (both tarsal and scleral) may accompany inflammatory changes of the tarsal margins or may occur as an isolated finding. Some clinicians have suggested that such conjunctival injection is one of the earliest signs of ocular rosacea and that it can even be a feature of frequent flushers who have a predisposition to rosacea or an early sign

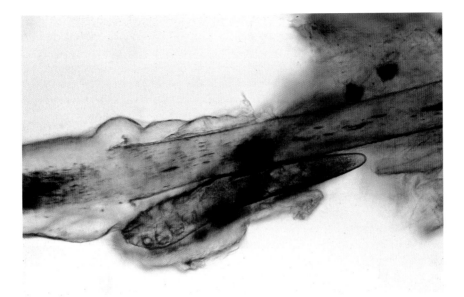

Figure 7   A lash which was plucked from the lid of the patient shown in fig 6 reveals a demodex mite encased in the keratin at the base of the lash.

of ocular rosacea in those with ETTR. Redness, irritation, and a discharge that causes the eyelids to stick together in the mornings may indicate the presence of conjunctivitis.

Chalazion (a cyst of the meibomian gland resulting from a blockage of the duct) gives rise to a relatively asymptomatic erythematous papulonodular swelling on the eyelid as seen in figures 3 and 5. Some patients with ocular rosacea get recurrent chalazia and if these become infected or inflamed they form large tender painful swellings within the eyelid called hordeola interna. Hordeolum externum (a focus of inflammation in one the glands of Zeiss) gives rise to a "stye" or small inflammatory pustule at the lid margin.

As indicated earlier, keratitis (usually a mild punctate epithelial keratitis involving the inferior cornea) can occur in patients with ocular rosacea and may be secondary to abnormalities in the composition of tear film and its breakup time. Neovascularisation of the cornea is rarely seen. A peripheral "spade-like" triangular infiltrate of the cornea with its base at the limbus is said to be characteristic, but its occurrence is rare. Uveitis, scleritis and episcleritis, and iritis are all fortunately rarely reported ocular manifestations of rosacea, but highlight the fact that all patients who complain of serious symptoms (pain, blurring of vision, photosensitivity, etc.) or persistent ocular symptoms in spite of treatment should be referred to an ophthalmologist for specialist attention.

Ocular rosacea may be graded as being mild (mild itch, dryness or grittiness of the eyes; fine scaling of lid margins; telangiectasia and erythema of lid margins; mild conjunctival injection), moderate (burning or sting of eyes;

crusting or irregularity of lid margins with erythema and edema; formation of chalazion or hordeolum), or severe (pain, photosensitivity, blurred vision, loss of eyelashes, severe conjunctival inflammation, corneal changes, scleritis or episcleritis, uveitis, iritis). Although ocular rosacea has been reported in childhood (5), it is very uncommon. It is difficult to confirm the validity of the diagnosis of OR in this age group because of the lack of specificity of the signs and symptoms and in the absence of any confirmatory test.

HISTOPATHOLOGY

The histopathological changes seen depend on the nature of the lesion studied. Thus, conjunctival and tarsal infiltration of lymphohisteocytic cells with bacterial elements and crusting may be seen in patients with blepharoconjunctivitis. Dilatation and obstruction of meibomian gland ducts with abnormal keratinisation (6) may be seen in those with meibomian gland dysfunction, while cystic degeneration with chronic inflammatory cells and possibly granuloma formation is seen in patients with chalazia.

DIFFERENTIAL DIAGNOSIS

When a patient who has evidence of cutaneous rosacea presents with ocular symptoms it should not be assumed that these are always linked with the skin disorder. As in any clinical situation, consideration should be given to the fact that the patient's eye complaints are an issue distinct from the skin disorder and in cases of doubt, the opinion of an ophthalmologist should be sought. Thus, meibomian cysts can be mistaken for a suppurative inflammation of the gland of Zeis (a stye) which usually points near the base of the cilia or a cyst of Moll which has a translucent appearance and is found at the lid margin in the region of an eyelash. Complaints of pain in the affected eye, photophobia, visual disturbance or any loss of vision, and persistence of any ocular symptoms after apparently adequate treatment measures are instituted should always prompt referral. The various ocular disorders that may be considered in the differential diagnosis of ocular rosacea fall into the specialist sphere of ophthalmology and are beyond the remit of this work.

> *"Cold tea is good when applied to hot eyelids"*
> As related to the author by a patient as a treatment for blepharritis secondary to OR.

MANAGEMENT

Most of the patients who present to the clinician with ocular rosacea have relatively mild disorders and can be treated with simple measures (Table 2). For those patients who complain of dryness of the eyes without evidence of inflammation, artificial

Table 2 Treatment of Ocular Rosacea

Therapy	Comment
Artificial tears	Frequently needed for "dry eyes" of ocular rosacea.
	Use several times daily.
Lid and lash hygiene	Using warm soaks or compresses.
	Can use saline or dilute baby shampoo lavage.
	Overnight creams soften scale and remove plugs from meibomian gland orifices.
Expression of Meibomian glands	Following hygiene gentle manual massage extrudes thickened wormlike secretions from glands.
Topical antibiotics	Effective treatment for infected blepharitis applied twice daily after lid hygiene.
	Fucidin, metronidazole/erythromycin/azelaic acid are main options.
Topical steroids	Use with caution. 1% hydrocortisone cream for blepharitis.
	May be used in antibiotic/steroid combination.
Tacrolimus/ cyclosporine	Insufficient evidence to know indications/role in therapy as yet.
Systemic antibiotics	As used for PPR.
	Minocycline, doxycycline, oxytetracycline, erythromycin commonly used.
	6–12 wk therapy.
	Response begins after 2 wk.
	Metronidazole used rarely.
	Relapse common after course of therapy completed.
Surgery	Incision and curettage for chalazion after eyelid everted.
	Required for keratitis if impending perforation.
Other therapies	Topical sulfur/zinc/icthymol preparations, hexachlorocyclohexane.
	Vitamin B_2 orally or parentally.
	Omega 3 fatty acid dietary supplementation.
	Topically applied cold tea or T tree oil.

tears are the preferred treatment. Cold winds exacerbate symptoms and wearing glasses or sunglasses can offer protection. When there is inflammation of the lashes or lid margins warm soaks or compresses, or commercially available eye scrubs help to settle the symptoms by removing the debris around the lashes and stimulating meibomian gland secretion. Eyelash and eyelid margin lavage can be carried out twice daily using a warm saline solution in an egg cup with a drop of baby shampoo added. A cotton-tipped applicator dipped in this solution can be used to brush the eyelids from the base to the ends (the upper lid with the eye closed and the lower lid with the lid pulled down). Manual expression of the meibomian glands daily to release the thickened yellowish secretions may be required in some patients and this will be facilitated by the prior lavage and removal of the material plugging the follicular orifices. If there are collaret's of keratin about the base of the lashes a cream applied to these over night helps to soften the keratin and facilitate its removal in the morning.

Bacterial infection of the lashes or lids usually appears as adherent yellow crusting or scaling. Topical fucidin or erythromycin cream or 1% metronidazole gel can be effective when applied twice daily in this situation. Other topical agents which have been used in the treatment of blepharitis in rosacea patients include niacinamide, azelaic acid, cyclosporine, and tacrolimus. Topical corticosteroids can be useful in reducing the inflammatory changes of the lid margins but should preferably be used under the supervision of an ophthalmologist because of their potential for side effects. In the past various preparations containing sulfur, zinc, and icthymol were used to treat the ocular symptoms of rosacea but the scientific evidence to support their use is lacking and they are no longer prescribed.

Systemic antibiotic therapy as used for PPR (see chap. 5) is an effective treatment of the inflammatory lesions of ocular rosacea. Their use is indicated in moderate or severe cases or in patients whose symptoms are unresponsive to topical therapy. Their mechanism of action in ocular rosacea is unclear. There is usually a delay in response to treatment of approximately 2 weeks so the patient should be cautioned not to expect immediate results. Relapse occurs in a significant proportion of patients after cessation of systemic antibiotic therapy so that repeated courses and/or maintenance of topical therapy is necessary to sustain remission. Thus minocycline 100 mg once or twice daily or doxycycline (either low "sub antimicrobial" dosages or 100 mg daily) for 6 weeks is usually well tolerated and improves the symptoms and signs of ocular rosacea in the majority of patients treated. Other antibiotics that can be helpful in the management of ocular rosacea include oxytetracycline 500 mg twice daily and erythromycin 500 mg twice daily for 6 weeks. Rarely metronidazole may be prescribed as a systemic medication, but its potential for adverse side effects limits its use to otherwise unresponsive cases. Isotretinoin, which is occasionally used to treat PPR or early PR can have an adverse effect on ocular rosacea due to its drying effect on the ocular secretions. This effect tends to compound the already dry eyes of the rosacea sufferer and the clinician should be alert to this potential effect. Sometimes, systemic corticosteroid therapy is required to control the more serious inflammatory ocular changes but the decision to administer these agents should be left to the ophthalmologist.

Surgical intervention may be required for chalazion (as these rarely undergo spontaneous resolution) or if serious keratitis evolves with potential for corneal melting.

KEY POINTS

- Ocular rosacea is common and often overlooked by the patient and clinician.
- Symptoms are usually mild and serious consequences of ocular rosacea are rare.

- Patients should use artificial tears and lid and lash hygiene techniques.
- Topical antibiotics can be helpful in mild cases of blepharitis.
- Systemic antibiotic treatment is usually effective for ocular rosacea but relapse is common.
- Pain, photophobia, or symptoms that persist in spite of therapy mandate referral to an ophthalmologist.

REFERENCES

1. Starr PAJ, Macdonald A. Oculocutaneous aspects of rosacea. Proc R Soc Med 1969; 62:9–11.
2. Quarterman MJ, Johnson DW, Abele DC, et al. Ocular rosacea: signs symptoms and tear studies before and after treatment with doxycycline. Arch Dermatol 1997; 133:49–54.
3. Gudmundsen KJ, O'Donnell BF, Powell FC. Schirmer testing for dry eyes in patients with rosacea. J Am Acad Dermatol 1992; 26:211–214.
4. Barton K, Monroy DC, Pflugfelder SC. Inflammatory cytokines in the tears of patients with ocular rosacea. Ophthalmology 1990; 104:1868–1874.
5. Chamaillard M, Mortemousque B, Boralevi F, et al. Cutaneous and ocular signs of childhood rosacea. Arch Dermatol 2008; 144:167–171.
6. To Kw, Hoffman RJ, Jakobiec FA. Excessive squamous hyperplasia of the Meibomian duct in acne rosacea. Arch Ophthalmology 1994; 112:160–161.

FURTHER READING

To learn more about the ocular changes that can be seen in patients with rosacea and the various approaches to their management the reader is advised to consult an up to date Ophthalmology text.

8

General Considerations

"Le traitement? C'est moi!"
Henri Gougerot

The response of a famous French dermatologist when asked what form of treatment was most effective for his patients. His reply emphasizes the importance of the patient's confidence in the treating physician to achieving good results in the management of skin disorders. Without confidence compliance will be poor.

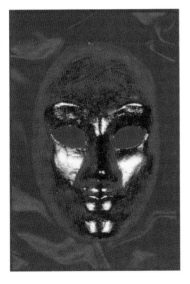

Figure 1   Patients who have severe rosacea often say that they feel that they are wearing a "mask of redness". They feel that people look at their red faces and do not see them as individuals. An understanding sympathetic approach to the management of their skin condition by the treating clinician is essential to win their confidence and to ensure compliance with suggested therapy.

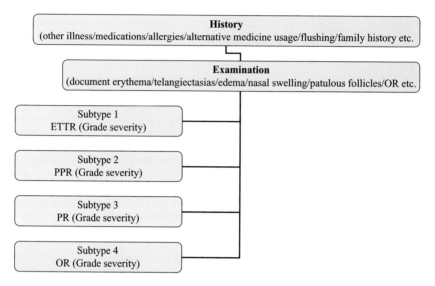

Algorithm 1   Approach to the patient suspected of having Rosacea.

The general approach to the patient suspected of having rosacea is summarized in Algorithm 1. Much of this has been covered in the previous chapters but is summarized here for convenience with some practical points relating to skin care, cosmetic cover, the correct application of topical medications, and the special considerations necessary in patients of color and those pregnant patients who suffer from rosacea.

DIAGNOSIS

As in any branch of medicine, the accuracy of the diagnosis is the fundamental and most important consideration in the approach to the patient with rosacea. This is based primarily on taking a thorough clinical history and performing a careful clinical examination. Because there is no laboratory test to confirm the clinical impression of rosacea, most investigations are undertaken in order to eliminate other possible diagnoses (see Figures 2 and 3).

(a) History

Although the physician may be able to make the diagnosis of rosacea within minutes of the patient entering the examination room, it is prudent and often informative to enquire into aspects of the patient's history that may explain the initiation of their complaint. For example, an underlying polycythemia may be responsible for a plethoric facies or the lack of response to previous therapy may be because the patient was applying a topical steroid cream to their face. In addition, the medication that a patient is taking may alter the expression of their disease

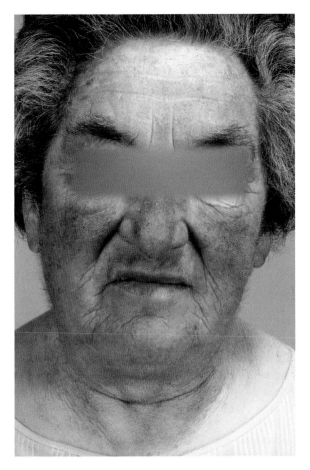

Figure 2 This older lady has facial erythema (with a cyanotic hue) and telangiectasias suggestive of ETTR. She complained of cold intolerance and had a puffy facial appearance and the dry appearing bushy gray hair. Appropriate serological tests established the diagnosis of hypothyroidism and replacement therapy was instituted.

(niacin used for its lipid lowering properties may exacerbate a tendency to flushing) or interact with therapy prescribed for rosacea (the absorption of tetracyclines may be affected by antacids used for heartburn).

Enquiry should be directed towards whether the patient is prone to flushing reactions. These symptoms will seldom be volunteered by the rosacea patients because they may not relate them to their cutaneous disorder. As discussed in chapter 2, many types of flushing reactions can be reduced by avoiding precipitating or exacerbating factors.

It is also wise to ask about the use of complementary or alternative medicines. Over 20% of rosacea patients use these (mostly herbal products) and may not

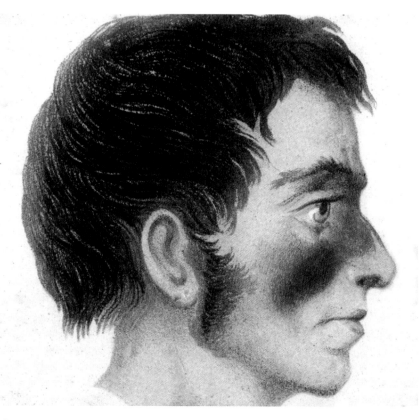

Figure 3   The young man who is shown here has striking malar and nasal erythema which could be mistaken for ETTR. However he has a thin emaciated appearance and was in fact suffering from the terminal stages of "phthisis" (pulmonary tuberculosis). This drawing was apparently made one week before his death.

spontaneously disclose this to the physician (1). These agents may interact with conventional medications that the physician prescribes. The roles of complementary and alternative medications in the management of rosacea have yet to be fully explored and some agents may well have a role to play in the management of aspects of rosacea. An example of the type of alternative treatment used by rosacea patients to treat redness and swelling of the face is the topical application of a chilled puree of cucumber. Cucumber (cucumis sativus) was mentioned as early as 1649 in Culpeppers text on Herbal Remedies as a treatment for facial redness. It has been reported to be effective by some patients. However it may be slightly irritant so caution is advised in its use. It is evident that stress management is important, especially in patients with a propensity to frequent flushing who often develop an anticipatory anxiety that certain social situations will provoke flushing. Meditation and relaxation techniques may be helpful in some of these patients.

Naturopathic dietary recommendations may be helpful in that they can enable the rosacea patient identify foods which flare their disease. The use of facial massage has been mentioned in the treatment of the persistent edema of rosacea. Massage should be carried carefully as it may initially exacerbate redness and cause discomfort. A non-scented moisturizing cream is first applied to the finger pulps which are then used to gently massage the skin in a rotatory movement beginning with the central region of the forehead and moving gradually outwards towards the temples. The same process is then used on the nose moving from the root to the alae nasi. Apparently the benefit of massage therapy may not be seen until several weeks of treatment have been institiuted. The role (if any) of reflexology and acupuncture in the management of rosacea is unknown.

Every patient with the cutaneous stigmata of rosacea should be questioned about eye symptoms, such as itchy, dry (contact lens intolerant), watery or frequently "bloodshot" eyes. Sometimes a history of recurrent sties or eyelid cyst removal will betray the underlying tendency to ocular rosacea. Many patients who say they have no problems with their eyes describe the use of significant quantities of eye drops each week.

It is also important to enquire if there is a family history of rosacea (approximately 10% of rosacea patients have a positive family history of the disease). A family history of rhinophyma may explain the intense anxiety in a patient who has only mild disease. Finally, the physician should document if the patient has previously been prescribed treatment for rosacea and what the response has been, and whether they have suffered any allergic reactions to medications in the past.

(b) Examination

Having taken a comprehensive history a close examination of the face (and any other areas that the patient says might be affected) should take place. It is important to document on the first visit if there are telangiectasias present, and if so their severity and distribution. The degree of facial erythema (mild, moderate, or severe) and its distribution, the presence and number of inflammatory lesions and whether there are ocular signs should also be documented. If edema or phymatous changes are present, these should also be recorded. When the physical examination is completed, the patient can be categorized as having one of the subtypes of rosacea (see Algorithm 1). This is helpful because it will guide the physician towards the appropriate treatment for that patient. In general, the patients' compliance with treatment is likely to be better if this is not unduly complex or intrusive on their daily routine. Thus, both oral and topical medications should be prescribed to be taken or applied once or twice daily at the same time if possible.

> *"The young physician starts life with twenty drugs for each disease. The old physician ends life with one drug for twenty diseases"*
> William Osler

APPLYING MEDICATIONS AND SKIN CARE

Patients should be encouraged to develop a nonirritating skin care routine that will ensure that the skin barrier is not compromised while at the same time debris, excess oil and surface organisms are removed. Facial skin should be cleansed twice daily with a moderate amount of tepid water splashed on to the skin surface. This is followed by the application of a fine lather of nonperfumated, uncolored gentle soap or soap-free cleanser. This is gently dabbed on to the skin surface using a moistened cotton wool pad or with the pads of the fingers. It is unnecessary and potentially irritating to rub the skin vigorously during the cleansing process. The skin is then blotted dry using a new cotton wool pad. Toweling should be avoided on the sensitive skin. If topical medications are to be applied, a rest period of up to 30 minutes should be taken after cleansing. This time period can be progressively reduced as the patient acclimatizes to the therapy. Medication should be applied as a fine film with a single movement of the finger pad from central to lateral face. Topical medications should be applied to the areas affected by rosacea, and not simply to the individual lesions. When the rosacea clears, the patient should continue to apply the medication to the same area to prevent relapses. It should not be massaged or rubbed vigorously into the skin. If a moisturizer or sun-block cream is to be used, these should be applied after the topical medication. The patient should be told to remember that the *"drugs have priority-they go on first!"* A moisturizer containing a sun-block agent will reduce the number of applications required to the skin and is often preferred by the patient. Excessive use of moisturizing creams (especially if combined with oily cleansers and absence of skin washing) can lead to the development of pityriasis folliculorum (see chapter 5). Greasy pomades should be avoided likewise as these can be associated with an acneform eruption on the forehead, especially if a tie is used to keep hair in place at night which occludes the pommade. Similarly, cleansing of the eyelid margins and application of topical medications and eye drops should be explained in simple terms to the patient to ensure that they understand the reasoning behind their use and to ensure compliance (see chapter 7).

COSMETIC ADVICE FOR THE ROSACEA PATIENT

Advice about improving the overall appearance of the patient's appearance is an important component of the management of rosacea. The use of cosmetic preparations by female patients with rosacea has recently been well reviewed by Draelos (2) and is summarized in Table 1. She advises rosacea patients to use cosmetics with few high quality pure ingredients. Cosmetics which compromise the skin barrier should be avoided. The use of a soft, dull, matte facial foundation containing a high sun-protective factor will mask erythema and reduce the damaging effects of ultraviolet light. All cosmetics are best applied with a brush to avoid the effect of friction on the sensitive facial skin. Sponges and face cloths are to be avoided. Similarly, eye shadow powders with a matte finish and of light brown color are best suited to the rosacea patient. Black, easily removed mascaras should

Table 1 Dos and Don'ts of Cosmetics for Patients with Rosacea (adapted from reference 2)

Do	Don't
Use powder cosmetics with a matte finish	Use cream/liquid cosmetics
Buy new cosmetics	Use old cosmetics
Wear light earth tones for eye shadow (tan, peach)	Wear deep eye shadows (Blue, purple, green, or pink)
Apply a separate sunblock after topical medication and before cosmetics	Use cosmetics containing perfume
Avoid cosmetics containing formaldehyde, propylene glycol, alcohol, toners, and palmitic and oleic acid	Purchase cosmetics with >10 ingredients
Use a brush applicator	Apply with a sponge or fingers
	Massage creams into the skin (unless edematous)
	Peeling "rejuvenating" agents
Use facial foundations of the powder/cream variety with a matte finish	Use light-reflective powders containing mica
Wear only black mascara	Use nail polish
Use pencil forms of eyeliner	

be used, as should regularly sharpened pencils to apply eyeliner to the lid margins. Waterproof eye cosmetics are best avoided as they require to be removed by solvents which can be irritating. Hair sprays should be used with caution avoiding any contact with the facial skin. If a patient is concerned that they may be allergic to a particular cosmetic preparation, patch testing should be carried out. The patient can alternatively instructed to carry out a "use test" (daily application for three days of the preparation in its normal form to a small area of facial skin—usually the lateral cheek) and to observe for any untoward reaction.

Men should also be counseled on the use of cosmetic products. Shaving with an electric razor is generally easier on the skin, but does not always produce a close enough shave. Skin cleansing gels, antibacterial soaps or those containing multiple particles, after shave lotions and astringents are not well tolerated by rosacea patients and can cause stinging and burning as well as heightening redness. Male patients are usually open to the use of a tinted sun-block cream, and tinted zinc oxide and even foundation are used by some men to diminish the appearance of erythema.

ROSACEA IN PREGNANCY AND IN PATIENTS WITH SKIN OF COLOR

Rosacea may appear for the first time or become exacerbated in patients who are pregnant. The management of the disorder during this phase of life can be difficult as it is best to avoid all systemic therapy. If considered essential in a patient with severe rosacea erythromycin given as outlined in chapter 5 is generally thought to be safe in pregnancy. Physicians are advised to consult with the obstetrician whose care the patient is under before commencing any such treatment. Tetracyclines and related drugs as well as both topical and systemic retinoids are contraindicated in the pregnant patient. The use of topical metronidazole and azelaic acid should be avoided. Topical erythromycin [applied twice daily for papulopustular rosacea (PPR)] is considered safe to prescribe to the pregnant patient. Rarely a mild topical steroid might be required for a short period to reduce the inflammatory component of PPR if this is troubling the patient severely.

Rosacea is uncommon in patients with skin of color (Fitzpatrick's skin types 4 to 6). However, when it occurs other considerations arise. Although the erythema is less visible in these individuals, they are aware of it and are prone to post inflammatory hyperpigmentation when papules and pustules resolve with therapy. In addition, they may have a propensity to developing a granulomatous response to inflammation which can result in more persistent, less responsive lesions. The use of topical retinoic acid in gradually increasing concentrations may help to treat the inflammatory lesions as well as reduce the post inflammatory effect. Azelaic acid as used for PPR also functions as a weak tyrosinase inhibitor (one of the enzymes central to the production of melanin) and so can be used as dual therapy to clear inflammatory lesions and reduce hyperpigmentation in those individuals who have rosacea and skin of color. Paradoxically, hypopigmentation may also result from rosacea in patients with darker skin. Topical calcineurin-inhibitors may help the hypopigmentation, but their use has been associated with rosaceiform eruptions, so caution should be exercised. It is important not to over-look advice on sun protection in patients who have darker skin as ultraviolet light may cause an exacerbation of their underlying erythema and promote skin damage.

DISCUSSING ROSACEA WITH PATIENTS

It is courteous to discuss with the patient what their concept of rosacea is. Important messages to convey are: rosacea is usually quite controllable and there are some factors that the patient can address in their lifestyles that may reduce the need for chronic medication usage. Patients should understand that while remissions can be long lived, there is no "cure" analogous to treating pneumonia with antibiotics. However, in some older patients the disorder seems to "burn itself out" and clear completely. Enquiry about seasonal exacerbations may allow the physician to develop a strategic plan with the patient to discontinue medications at certain times when the disorder is likely to be in remission. Many rosacea sufferers are concerned about the progression of the condition to culminate in disfiguring rhinophyma. Patients can be reassured that this outcome is quite rare, and female patients further consoled by the fact that the condition occurs almost exclusively in males! The earliest sign of rhinophyma (patulous follicles) should be sought and recorded on the patients first and subsequent visits. The absence of such can indicated as reassurance that this eventuality is unlikely. It is also helpful to tell the patient that at least two to three follow-up visits will be required to ensure that the treatment prescribed is effective and to determine if it can be reduced or discontinued.

ADDRESSING THE SOCIAL STIGMA OF ROSACEA

We have already mentioned the particular place that the patient with rosacea occupies within dermatology. Not only do they have a bright red skin disorder that is highly visible on the central face, are prone to blushing and have soreness and inflammation of their eyes, but they are also stigmatized by their disease (Fig 1). The unspoken implication of their rash to many of the people is that that they are abusing alcohol. This is the reason we applied the term "The Curse of the Celts" to this disorder in order encapsulate the tendency for the disorder to occur in individuals of Celtic origin together with the implied social stigma of excessive alcohol intake. It is therefore important to address this issue directly with the patient and to reassure them that this putative association is not valid. Many patients will appreciate being directed to appropriate Web sites for additional information about rosacea such as that of the American Academy of Dermatology—www.aad.com; the European Academy of Dermatology and Venereology—www.eadv.org; or the British Association of Dermatology—www.bad.org.uk. In addition, there are patient support groups in many countries. Probably the best-known of these is being the National Rosacea Society (NRS) of the United States which can be contacted at www.nrs.com. Patient support groups can play an important role in the dissemination of appropriate information, conducting surveys of members on issues relating to their disease, and collecting and distributing funds for research. In this regard, the NRS should be credited for funding research in several centers throughout the world (including in this authors laboratory) and for stimulating interest in rosacea.

By accessing information in this way and interacting with patient support groups the feeling of isolation that many patients experience when they develop rosacea can be reduced significantly.

A POSITIVE OUTLOOK

Although rosacea is unsightly and unpleasant for the patient in many ways, medical treatment in the majority of patients will bring a very significant improvement in their skin condition. There is active research being pursued in several countries that is likely to provide insight into its etiology and pathogenesis and provide for improved treatment modalities in the future. These positive facts should be emphasized to the patient at the outset of their therapy, as it is important to have an optimistic approach to improve compliance.

When a diagnosis of rosacea is made and the correct treatment instituted the improvement not only in the patients skin condition, but also in their demeanor and degree of social relaxation can be very rewarding for both the physician and patient alike Figures 4 and 5.

In its most severe form can have a devastating effect on the individual. It is hoped that this book will help to improvement patient care possibly progression of severity.

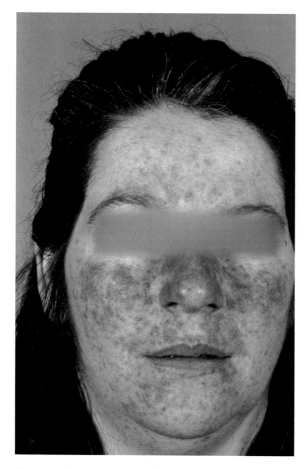

Figure 4   This young lady had severe PPR which caused much distress and greatly inhibited social interaction.

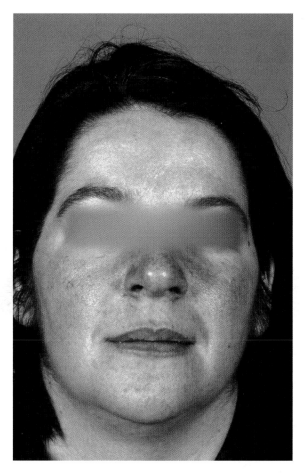

Figure 5 Following a 6-week course of low dose doxycylcline therapy and with topical azelaic acid cream applied twice daily, the skin condition has improved markedly. The patient appears relaxed and was able to function socially in a normal fashion again. Note the absence of any residual scarring following clearing of the inflammatory lesions.

KEY POINTS

- The history and clinical examination are crucial to the evaluation of a patient suspected of having rosacea
- Having made the diagnosis classify the patient according to subtype and grade the severity
- Be aware that the patient may be using alternative treatments for their skin condition.

- Advise the patient how to apply topical therapies to get the best results from treatment
- Cosmetic advise is important for both male and female patients with rosacea
- In pregnancy treatment choices are limited but topical erythromycin can be helpful
- Patients with skin of color are more prone to granulomatous skin lesions and may develop postinflammatory hyperpigmentation.
- Discuss the disease and its physical and social impact with patients. Refer them to an appropriate information source if they wish to enquire further.

REFERENCES

1. McAleer M, Powell FC. Herbal medicine usage in rosacea. Brit J Dermatol 2008. 158:1134–1135.
2. Draelos ZD. Treating beyond the histology of rosacea. Cutis 2004; 74(suppl 35):28–31.

Index